Rhythmical Massage

AS INDICATED BY ITA WEGMAN, M.D.

Margarethe Hauschka, M.D.

translated by L.D. Monges

MERCURY PRESS

Copyright © 1990 by Schule Für Künstlerische Therapie, Boll, Germany

First English Edition, Rudolf Steiner Press, London 1979
Second Revised English Edition, Mercury Press, Spring Valley 1990
Third Revised English Edition, Mercury Press, Spring Valley 1991

ISBN 978-1-957569-21-5

Authorized translation from the German:
Rhythmische Massage nach Dr. Ita Wegman
Schule Für Künstlerische Therapie, Boll, Germany

MERCURY PRESS
an imprint of SteinerBooks
www.steinerbooks.org

CONTENTS

Foreword

PART ONE
The Knowledge Underlying the Method

1. The History of Massage 1
2. The Members of Man's Being 8
3. The Threefold Membering of the Human Organism 11
4. The Water Organism 16
5. The Air Organism 20
6. The Warmth Organism 23
7. Nerve and Blood 29
8. Circulation and Heart 32
9. Metamorphoses of the Skeleton 36
10. The Muscle System 42
11. The Inner World System 49
12. The Skin 53

PART TWO
Rhythmical Massage according to Dr. Ita Wegman

13. Development and Elaboration 60
14. Harmony and Disharmony of the Members of Man's Being 62
15. The Law of Polarity in Massage 67
16. The Qualities of Grip 73
17. The Use and Quality of Oils in Rhythmical Massage 78
18. Rhythm 81
19. The Lemniscate and the Pentagram 85
20. The Basic Forms 88

PART THREE
The Application of Rhythmical Massage

21. Embrocations of the Organs 102
22. The Spinal Column and its Treatment 111
23. Indications for the Treatment of Specific Condtions 116
    1. General Effects of Rhythmical Massage 116
    2. Bronchial Asthma 117
    3. Angina Pectoris and Related Conditions 117
    4. Disturbances in Arterial Blood Supply 118
    5. Venous Symptom Complex 119
    6. Disturbances of Sleep 120

    7. *Headaches of Various Origins* 121
    8. *Constipation* 122
    9. *Rheumatic Diseases* 123
   10. *Periarthritis of the Shoulder Joint* 124
   11. *After-Treatment of Fractures* 124
   12. *Neuritis* 125
   13. *Poliomyelitis and Paralysis of Other Genesis* 125
   14. *Degenerative Illnesses of the Nervous System* 126
   15. *Treatment of Cancer Patients* 127
   16. *Rhythmical Massage in Curative Education* 128
   17. *Rhythmical Massage in Psychiatry* 130
24. Therapeutic Technique 132
25. The Hand 134

FOREWORD

This book is presented by request of the practising masseurs and prescribing medical doctors who have worked for decades with the Rhythmical Massage developed by Dr. Ita Wegman. Because of its special effect they will no longer do without this method. New viewpoints arising when the field of massage is worked through on the basis of Rudolf Steiner's spiritual-scientific knowledge of man are presented.

I had to consider as my special domain of work the elaboration of Rhythmical Massage under the direction of Dr. Ita Wegman (Arlesheim, Switzerland) as well as the further development of this method during the past three decades. Since I must introduce this method of healing into the sphere of spiritual-scientific medicine, this book will contain more than an isolated description of this method of massage. Rhythmical Massage does not present a ready-made dogmatic system. First, the chief phenomena that appear in this domain will be shown. Understanding of these will be aided by the concepts of the Goetheanistic science of nature which takes hold of the element of the living. There are fundamental forms suited to the body that have to be learned. The actual treatments are metamorphoses of these basic forms, or even enhancements in the Goethean sense, and grow out of them as completely individual actions. The actual curative massage is an art—as is healing in general—and no technique, even though the master of a technique of a special nature forms the basis, as is the case in every art. Of like importance is the expanded knowledge of man's body, soul, and spirit, and of the healthy or unhealthy interplay of these principles. Although there is an extended literature dealing with these facts in the lectures of Rudolf Steiner or in the works of his students, I feel it my duty to present again the spiritual-scientific knowledge of man, and above all, the members of man's being insofar as it is necessary for the domain of massage, in order to make this book generally comprehensible without any preconceptions.

It presupposes the reader's readiness to be open to the spiritual-scientific viewpoints without prejudice.

Nobody, however, should presume that Rhythmical Massage may be learned solely from this book. No art can be learned from books. There must be places where this massage is practised and where the students through sensitive perception and imitation can take hold of the nature of Rhythmical Massage.

This book is written for the assistant of the medical doctor and in its presentation avoids the purely medical problems and questions, although a general comprehension of the nature of illnesses must be present in the non-medical professions of healing. The boundary cannot be sharply drawn.

To all those who have contributed to the publication of this book I should like to express my most cordial thanks. This gratitude extends to many people, for it has been a long process of human encounters and experience that has given me the possibility of presenting this large field in surveyable and pictorial form.

Boll, March 1972
Dr. Margarethe Hauschka

PART ONE

THE KNOWLEDGE UNDERLYING THE METHOD

1.

THE HISTORY OF MASSAGE

Consideration of the history of massage may broaden the outlook upon the entire domain of healing methods which change in the course of time. It is one field in the overall history of medicine described by Rudolf Steiner as accompanying the change of consciousness of mankind. Every epoch of time has different thoughts about the connection of man with the world, about illness, death, and healing. What we consider today to be the only reality, was for times past the great illusion, 'maya.' And what man experienced spiritually in earlier ages, in other states of consciousness, as essential being, was the 'reality' upon which matters depended. Rudolf Steiner described in detail in his fundamental book *An Outline of Occult Science* the gradual descent from the consciousness of vision throughout the ancient cultures down to our sensory consciousness limited to the physical world. Thus also medicine gradually transformed its spiritual healing methods practised in the mysteries of antiquity, after the latter's decay, into a treatment of the physical body along with substances of nature and finally with synthetic substances designated by Rudolf Steiner in this connection as 'sub-nature.' This transformation took place slowly through millennia. It can, however, be demonstrated by a striking phenomena.

If we observe the history of mankind in its totality as far as the Mystery of Golgotha, it presents the history of the gradual descent of the soul and spirit of man into the physical body.

Only between the third and second millenia B.C. did those who were the carriers of culture at that time begin to identify with the physical body instead of experiencing it as merely a sheath. While up to that time the continuity of life in the spirit from pre-earthly existence through the earth life into the time after death was a self-evident conviction, there now began the uncertainty about the whereabouts of the soul after death. Rudolf Steiner shows how in the 'Epic of Gilgamesh' this ruler of peoples, after the death of his friend Eabani, in desperate uncertainty about the latter's whereabouts, journeys far toward the West in order to be instructed in the last branches of the Hibernian Mysteries about the secrets of death and the indestructibility of the spirit.

Prior to this time all methods of healing, such as the Egyptian 'temple sleep,' were purely spiritual procedures. Trained priest-physicians were able to direct the souls of the ill in the spiritual world, while in sleep they were lifted out of the body, enabling them to perceive the 'archetype of health' revered as Isis insofar as she represents the image of the divine world soul, the pure archetype of the human soul before the fall of mankind. Perceiving her, the ill person experienced the correction in the spirit and in reawakening carried the healing impulses into the body. We must imagine here that in ancient times the soul possessed much more power over the physical body and was able really to transform it according to the prototype received in the healing sleep. Today such healing methods are no longer effective, because the physical bodies have hardened.

In prehistoric ages, the healing procedures for the body (with the exception of the treatment of wounds) bore the character of preparation and purification belonging to the temple rituals. Later on, the inner organs of the body were investigated, not in the sense of our present-day anatomy, but as an image of the macrocosm. 'Above, everything is as below' was the profound rule of Hermes.

The next stage may be observed in the Greek culture. It is still the soul whose paths are pursued, and the physician is still the priest-physician and healing is a temple ritual. It is Hippocrates who closes the Mysteries and begins to work in the outer world, founding exoteric medicine. In early Greece we still find the Mysteries of Aeskulapios which are of special interest because they clearly show the transition of the ancient purely spiritual methods to a therapy bound to the body.

In this short presentation I refer to an article by Walter Johannes Stein, which appeared in the magazine *Natura*, Volume 1, 1926/27. Aeskulapios was regarded as a son of Apollo. The Greeks saw in him a kind of Saviour, for they said of him 'Aeskulapios makes light the burden of those who are oppressed and suffering,' and they derived his name from *Askeles* (exhausted) and *Epios* (healing). In the body grotto of Aeskulapios after the necessary purifications the sick were laid to sleep as a lamb's skin, and the priest- physician observed their dreams. Here we find in a wondrous way the transition from the ancient body-free therapy to the body-bound therapy. In sleep the soul partially releases itself from its organic connections; we therefore lose consciousness in sleep. An in-between state arises which manifests as dream. If the soul is more strongly bound to the body, the patient dreams of his illness. The dream symbolizes his ailments, which even today is a well-known phenomenon. But when in deep sleep the soul was able to spread out into the cosmos, it was possible for man to experience his remedy in sleep. The body-free part of the soul dips down in sleep into the spiritual element of nature. The spiritual in nature is part of the Isis force, if we want to use the Egyptian image once more. The world soul also ensouls nature, the world body.—If now the soul of the sleeper looks back upon the sick body, the wish arises in it to cure the body, and it finds the remedy in nature. History reports such dreams in connection with Alexander the Great and others. The priests of Aeskulapios were trained in relating the macrocosm to the microcosm, man. They were able to trace the soul, on awakening, into the sick organ and thus attained a knowledge about the connection of nature substances with sick organs. Here the swing of the pendulum begins between diagnosis and therapy. Out of these sources Hippocrates drew his wisdom. For his later doctrine of the body fluids is also based upon the knowledge concerning the various ways in which the soul embeds itself into the bodily processes.

In order to understand better how man at that time conceived of his connection with nature I quote a passage from Walter Johannes Stein's article. He writes: 'Thus Aeskulapios is justified in using the wand of Mercury, the rod with snakes which the God Mercury received from Apollo and with which he is able to put to sleep or to awaken, that is, to bind or to loosen spirit and soul. Mercury was the spiritual teacher in all the ancient Mysteries of Healing; he was not an abstraction but a real spiritual being from whom the initiated priest-physician received his instruction.'

But evolution proceeded, and this meant: the spiritual world closed, man took over the ancient wisdom as tradition of the temple localities which gradually degenerated.

For us, the most important personality of antiquity is the physician Hippocrates. If it was stated that Hippocrates began to heal with substances, we must not conceive of this in the modern sense, nor must we think that no substances at all were used. Yet the points of view were different. The relationship of the soul-spiritual to the bodily was always emphasized. It must be noted that this short retrospect upon ancient methods does not claim completeness. It endeavors only to show the direction in which the art of healing metamorphosed. With the descending evolution of mankind's consciousness it developed gradually more and more downward into the perception of matter alone, and in future it will again transform itself in an ascending direction towards the spirit.

In the Greek age, at this special point of descending evolution, the nature of massage as well as of gymnastics finds its purest presentation. Here lie the fundamental principles. For the Greeks knew that the harmonious insertion of the soul into the body may best be effected through active and passive motion. In order to comprehend this we must occupy ourselves more closely with Greek consciousness. At that time a kind of equilibrium had been brought about in the relationship of the soul between the bodily and the spiritual world. The Greek, at the culmination of his culture, was a harmonious being between heaven and earth. According to his conviction, his Gods descended into his temples upon the sunlit surface of the earth. For the Egyptians the center of gravity of mankind's feeling still existed in the supersensible, and only the life after death promised them the complete fulfillment of their humanness; that is, the union with Osiris; indeed, actually becoming Osiris. But the Greeks lived in a very different cultural mood. Their soul joyfully took hold through the body of the surrounding, earthly world; they wanted to make their spirit active in the here and now, in serenity. The often quoted saying: 'Rather a beggar in the sunshine than a king in the realm of the shades' testifies to the waning intimacy with the spiritual world after death.

In this Greek age the soul wished to feel well in the body, it wanted to develop the body to its highest blossom, but not to perish in it and deny the spirit. The soul was not to forget its stellar origin but to shape the body harmoniously according to laws of the stars; it was to bring about circulation of the fluids and motion of the limbs according to heavenly laws. The Greek felt the impulses of Mars when he stepped forth courageously, the rulership of Venus when his body moved artistically. Saturn gave the inclination to sleep, Jupiter bestowed thought movement and sculptural force. It is thus not astonishing that Greek art produced those unique sculptures through which we sense how a 'star soul' shapes living fluids into the divine forms of bodily substance. The Greek expresses the human form in such a way that the highest principle, the spirit—today called the 'I' or ego—rules and brings everything into harmonious order. The horses obey the reins of the charioteer. The spirit and soul bestow what Goethe called noble simplicity and quiet grandeur, two qualities which mark all Greek works of art.

At that time gymnastics and massage came into existence in order to influence the body-soul equilibrium, enabling the body to become a healthy instrument for the cultural task of the Greeks. The care of the body, through active and passive motion, had a universal educational and therapeutic character. It was practised in the gymnasiums which were at first always linked with the temple sanctuaries. Naturally, later on they emancipated themselves from the temples, as did the entire art of healing.

The directives of Hippocrates that have come down to us—I quote them from Kirchhoff's book on massage—are really intelligible only against this background.

They are:
    Strong rubbing stabilizes (rubbing means massaging).
    Slight rubbing loosens.
    Much rubbing makes parts disappear.
    Moderate rubbing makes parts grow.

This way of treating the body, the physiological basis of which will be described later on, still rests upon the insight that the penetration of the soul into the body stimulates from inside the unconscious life processes (growth, tonus, gland activity) in the same way that they are stimulated in the plant from outside, from the cosmos. These processes do not produce consciousness. The formation of consciousness can only take place upon the basis of breaking down processes. Heightening of body consciousness through much rubbing makes the parts; i.e., body substance, disappear, as Hippocrates states.

The Greeks, with their doctrine of body fluids and their Aristotelian theory of the elements which transmit the cosmic to the earth and to man, still practised this art of gymnastics and massage by viewing at the same time the influences of these cosmic elements. Rudolf Steiner points out that the Athenians took into account in their exercises the sun, the shadows, and the outer conditions of air, thus producing harmonious and eloquent natures, open to the outer world. In contrast, the Spartans, disregarding these meteorological conditions, through rigorous hardening of the body (as we would say today), driving the soul inward, produced terse, hardened, but also at times profound natures. These differences throw a light upon the fact that the type of bodily care affects the body-soul relationship and thereby also the formation of consciousness of an epoch.

After the Mysteries, in which human beings were brought to the beholding of spiritual connections, had been closed, the ancient wisdom was imparted to posterity through tradition. Gradually came the treatment of the physical body alone. The teachings of Hippocrates, who himself was still a pupil of the Mysteries, proved true in practice during long periods. Proof of this was his own, almost godlike, reputation and the reputation of his great pupils. Hippocratic knowledge carried through, as it were, the whole of Roman history. Indeed, it radiated far into the Middle Ages. In Rome especially, these teachings fell upon fertile ground. Most physicians were Greeks. A great number of them called themselves Asclepiades, after Aeskulapios, documenting thereby the origin of their wisdom and methods. Galen's numerous writings in which he elaborated the details of Hippocratic teaching, have been preserved up to our time. The elements warmth, air and water, and also mud (earth) still play a role greater than that of remedies. Also purging and bleeding are measures that influence the circulation into which, through the breath, the soul dips down creating living pulsation. Centuries later the mystery knowledge of Hippocrates is still effective and gives a deeper meaning to concepts which today we use only materialistically and abstractly. Thus the teaching about the elements which Aristotle gave to his pupil Alexander the Great is something entirely different from our conception of aggregate conditions. Fire, water, air, and earth were understood to be conditions of the world of substances, each of which mediated a different cosmic entity to the earth or the physical body. A special chapter of this book will be dedicated to this doctrine of the elements.

After the Mystery of Golgotha, Christianity rising from the catacombs brought about a new era in history and culture. The ancient pagan wisdom was persecuted, the body was considered sinful and emphasis was laid on the soul which strove for a unison with Christ in the beyond, mindful of the words 'My realm is not of this world.' These first Christian centuries were filled with the urge to free the soul again from the fetters of the sinful body. The Mystery of Golgotha had, indeed, brought the turning point for the evolution of all mankind; into the descending phase of evolution the seed was sown for its transformation into an ascending evolution. Today we no longer have an adequate conception of the intensity of this impulse of the martyrs and conquerors of death in the first centuries A.D. But their striving, directed exclusively toward the beyond, made the ancient insights concerning the care of the body gradually disappear. In addition, in the Eighth and Ninth Centuries a completely new impulse out of the Arabian world had entered science. Medicine began to occupy itself exclusively with research into the sensory facts. Thus already in the Middle Ages the corpse and no longer the living human being became the basis of further development. The age of tradition was at an end. The new age of empiricism began. The therapies with the natural remedies of the elements disappeared from the view of the highly educated physicians trained in the universities of Arabian orientation.

After a comparatively long pause people began to concern themselves once more with the domain of body care in the Eighteenth and Nineteenth Centuries. We may disregard the efforts to invigorate youth through athletics as practised in Prussia by the founder of German gymnastics, Friedrich Ludwig Jahn, because this was an impulse of martial, not mercurial character. The situation was different in Sweden where at the beginning of the Nineteenth Century a man appeared who gave to gymnastics and massage a new world-wide reputation. His name was Per Henrik Ling. He brought about a turning point in the history of massage and we must consider him more closely. It is significant that he was not a physician. Son of a parson and orphaned at a young age, he first turned to theology and later became a tutor in Germany. After having participated as an officer in several campaigns and returning with a severe rheumatic ailment, he is reported to have cured himself by fencing exercises. He turned his whole interest to the field of gymnastics and massage after having experienced in his own body the beneficial effect of these measures. Perceived primarily as a means of education, but also as prophylactic and direct therapy for various diseases, he elaborated a system of simple and duplicated movements that must be considered as a new creation in this field. In the course of his work he distinguished between army drill, pedagogic, medical, and aesthetic gymnastics. In his textbook of massage and curative gymnastics (*Handbuch der Massage und Heilgymnastik*) Dr. Franz Kirchberg characterizes Ling's concept of life: 'He considered life to consist of the collaboration of three basic forms, the dynamic, the chemical, and the mechanical, which bring about through their interaction the variety of life's phenomena'. This conception appears like a faded recollection of ancient wisdom which knew that behind all phenomena of life there is to be found a cooperation of forces that are designated in modern Spiritual Science with the expressions *astral* (dynamic), *etheric* (chemical-biological) and *physical* (mechanical). To be sure, there is no conformity of concepts, but only a last echo of a forgotten melody. After overcoming enormous difficulties, Per Henrik Ling succeeded in 1813 in founding a state institute in Stockholm. This institute gained world-wide renown. Students from many countries came to Sweden. Ling worked for twenty-six years at this place and trained countless students. Swedish curative gymnastics and massage have become generally known concepts.

Ling's successors, however, in accordance with the tendencies of the times, began to give the rather complicated system a technical slant. Nevertheless, his great indications continued to be effective. Present-day Swedish massage is a combination of the elements of Ling's method and the work of the Dutch physician Mezger who was active in Amsterdam in the second half of the Nineteenth Century, and was much sought after because of his great success. He handed on the old manipulations and introduced massage to modern medicine.

Today medicine has become much more specialized, but also more materialistic, and, speaking with Goethe, we hold in our hand the parts, but the spiritual connection threatens to be lost. There exist a whole series of special methods that proceed from the individual systems of the body, from anatomical-physiological points of view that correspond to the modern conception of bodily activities as the only reality.

But now Rudolf Steiner's image of man, which he describes in Spiritual Science, can give a basis upon which the comprehensive field of active and passive motion can be newly viewed. In the following chapters we shall attempt to describe as much of it as is necessary for an understanding of the interplay between the soul-spiritual parts of man with the physical-bodily parts. This can only be a sketch. A large body of literature is available for a deeper study.

2.

THE MEMBERS OF MAN'S BEING

Knowledge of man's body, soul and spirit and of the way these members interweave is one of the necessary requirements for the purposes of this book because the normal or abnormal; i.e. disturbed, interplay of these 'members of man's being,' as Rudolf Steiner calls the higher principles, determines health and illness.

Since sufficient literature exists concerning exact spiritual-scientific concepts of these members, I shall limit myself to a short presentation of the conditions important for our theme. The presentation of the members of man's being in the book *Fundamentals of Therapy*, is specially suited for the medical field. This was Rudolf Steiner's last publication and he worked on it in collaboration with Dr. Ita Wegman.

The *physical body*, in the narrower sense, is the material body which science has investigated thoroughly. It contains everything that is to be found in the anatomical textbooks. In addition, it consists of the aggregate states of the elements earth, water, air, and fire, as already taught by Aristotle. It is fourfold, consisting of the solid, 'earthly,' body, the fluid body, the airy, gaseous body and the warmth body.

If, however, the higher principles, life, soul, and spirit, were not to intervene through their media, water, air and fire—through the fluid, aeriform, and heat principles, the physical body alone would be the corpse that is at once dissolved by the earth's forces when the higher principles have left it.

The fact that we live we owe to the first supersensible member of man's being; namely, to the *life* or *ether body*, also called formative force body, which with its forces permeates the water organism of man and is rooted in it.

We owe the fact that we are soul beings to the *soul body* or *astral body* which unites with the physical body through the air element. Let us remember the Biblical words: 'And God breathed into his nostrils the breath of life.' Through breathing the astral body unites with the physical body.

Finally, the spirit permeation with the force of our individuality takes place through the *ego*, the 'I,' which is not merely a point but a spiritual organism. This ego is bound up with our warmth organism and demands for man the characteristic temperature of 37 degrees C.

Physical body, ether body, astral body, and *ego* thus bring forth the interplay that stands before us as the whole human being. Concerning these names of the members of man's being Rudolf Steiner says in the book mentioned above that the names were given in connection with the ancient instinctive notions of these facts which today, however, are no longer of cognitive value when compared with the clear conceptions of the scientist of the spirit. Yet, if we wish to designate something, we need names.

The word 'etheric' points to delicate substantiality, to lightness in contrast to the heaviness of all physical substances. The word 'astral' shows the connection of all soul forces with the forces of the stellar world, the astra. And the 'I,' the ego designates the innermost spiritual kernel of the entelechy man. Therefore the remarkable word 'I' can never approach me from outside if it intends to designate me.

The forces radiating from the inner regions of the earth, the forces of gravity, work only upon the solid, mineral body. This would not live if it did not contain a *fluid* man into which is inserted the first supersensible body, the ether or life body. It is an individually organized complex of forces just as the physical body is a complex of substances. The ether body is the builder and former of the physical body, for the latter is shaped according to cosmic laws which the ether body provides. The functional within the physical form, the sum total of growth and life processes, is the ether body's domain. The physical forms are to be considered the coagulated result of the growth and formative forces of this ether body. The forces radiating from the cosmos work upon the ether body; they are the opposite of the earth forces and raise the mineral substances into life. Man possesses the ether body in common with the plant world; but his is more highly organized through the addition of soul and spirit.

The living body becomes ensouled through the development of a breathing system, that is to say, through the insertion of an *air body* of its own. Through the element 'air,' through the gaseous state of substances, soul-astral forces are able to take hold of the physical body. The quality of the soul is at home in the starry cosmos. This truth was acknowledged and experienced in the ancient cultures as self-evident. We owe to the astral body motion and consciousness, the capacities that distinguish us from the plant and which we share with the animals. Man has an entirely individual soul-astral body which takes hold of the air man and irradiates his whole nature. The expression 'astral body' is more comprehensive for the reason that we usually understand by the word 'soul' only the conscious part of this soul body, whereas the soul forces that have dipped down into the body and are bound to it also belong to it.

Finally, the physical body possesses a *warmth man*, an organized interconnected warmth body, the investigation of which has begun today through most delicate measurements of temperature. This warmth organism is the bearer of our spiritual individuality, permeates all previously described organisms, and is anchored in the blood.

Thus the bodily basis of a complete human personality is the fourfold physical body. The ether body, anchored in the fluid element, plays the role of mediator between the soul-spiritual and the physical-bodily. To take into account this body will be the prime task of an expanded art of healing.

The following will further lead to an understanding of the character of the members of man's being. Man is organized out of the spiritual from above downward. The spirit has primacy. The *ego*, then, is the *unity* that includes everything. The element of warmth or fire permeating everything is closest to the unity. The *soul-astral* is organized upon polarity; *duality*, with all its phenomena such as reflection, contrast, and so on, belongs to the astral world. Every soul quality has its opposite, the two basic forces are sympathy and antipathy in the objective, not merely subjective sense.

The *triad* belongs to the domain of the *etheric formative forces*, the functional is always a balance between two poles. Functions take place between two poles or polarities. The first consideration of this character of the etheric body is the concept of the functional threefold membering of the human organism.

The introduction of this concept through Rudolf Steiner is of unprecedented import. We need not wonder that the idea of the threefold membering was the result of thirty years' work of research, as Rudolf Steiner states in 1917 in the appendix to the first edition of his book *Von Seelenrätseln* (*Riddles of the Soul*).*

Finally, the physical body; that is, the effectiveness of forces acting purely physically in space, is *fourfold*. Here everything is ordered according to the four directions of space. The needle of the magnet points to the North. We orient ourselves on earth according to the four directions of space. Substances may appear in four forms of existence: solid, fluid, gaseous, warm.

It is not possible in this book to enter in more detail upon the history of creation and the evolution of mankind that would show the development of the members of man's being and which describes the descent out of spiritual states into matter and contains the view into the future ascent. The Mystery of Golgotha forms the nadir, but simultaneously the turning point, the unique central event of the whole earth evolution of mankind.

Whoever wishes to heal in the sense of spiritual-scientific medicine, will do well to enlarge his basis of knowledge again and again through the works of Rudolf Steiner.

In the subsequent chapters a brief foundation will be laid for these studies of the spiritual-scientific knowledge of man in its most important thoughts and phenomena.

---

* Rudolf Steiner Verlag, Dornach, 1960. Parts of this book are translated in *The Case for Anthroposophy*, Rudolf Steiner Press, London.

3.

THE THREEFOLD MEMBERING OF THE HUMAN ORGANISM

The functional threefold membering of the human organism, first described by Rudolf Steiner in 1917 in his book *Riddles of the Soul*, is the kernel of the new image of man.

We observe in man the *nerve-sense system* that has its center in the head but is present everywhere. Its processes constitute the bodily support of the conscious life of thinking.

The *rhythmical system* that has its organs in the chest but is also extended over the entire human being since it contains breathing and circulation in its finest ramifications, is the bodily support of the life of feeling.

And the *metabolic system*, that has its center in the lower man, is the bodily support of the life of will. Today, the nerve system is considered responsible for all three functions, but for the execution of a visualized act of will we need the basis of a metabolic process that produces heat, for we may be able to think the movement but are not able to carry it out. The basis of certain restrictions of will are delicate disturbances of metabolism. This life of metabolism continues on into the organs of movement; therefore Rudolf Steiner uses the expression metabolic-limb system. This is the counterpart of the fact that the nerve system is preceded by the sense system; i.e., sense-nerve system. Both are in a polar relationship. In the senses the effects of the outer world penetrate into us; they are inlets through which we allow the qualities of the outer world to enter us, such as light, color, tone, and so on. Through the limbs, however, we penetrate beyond ourselves into the outer world, changing it. The limbs are protrusions, as it were. If one considers the body of man as instrument of the soul, one must base it on this functional threefold membering. For the body as a whole is the instrument of soul and spirit which wish to move on the earth by thinking, feeling, and willing in order to fulfill the tasks of their eternal being.

The next most important knowledge flowing from the threefold membering is the insight that the metabolic processes are of upbuilding character whereas their polar opposite, the nerve-sense processes, are destructive. The forming of consciousness does not take place as a continuation of the upbuilding processes of the organism. Quite to the contrary, life must be sacrificed for consciousness. Consciousness-ness-bearing processes are death processes.

The rhythmical processes of the middle system create the healthy balance in life; they are harmonizing processes. Health is the biological equilibrium produced and maintained through a strong middle system, an equilibrium between the nourishing and reproductive processes of upbuilding that are only able to produce a sleep consciousness as in the plant, and the destructive breakdown processes of the nerve-sense system which, however, are accompanied by consciousness.

From this observation it becomes evident that massage must be rhythmical in order to strengthen the forces of the balancing system.

Once we have understood the polarity of the life of thought and the life of will also in regard to their bodily bases, the next step will be to seek the reason for this in the interplay of the four members of man's being, which is completely polaric in these domains.

For the comprehension of massage the very complicated relationships can be brought to a simple common denominator, using the following drawing.

In order to show the interplay of the members of man's being we can present their functional relationships through the following curves.

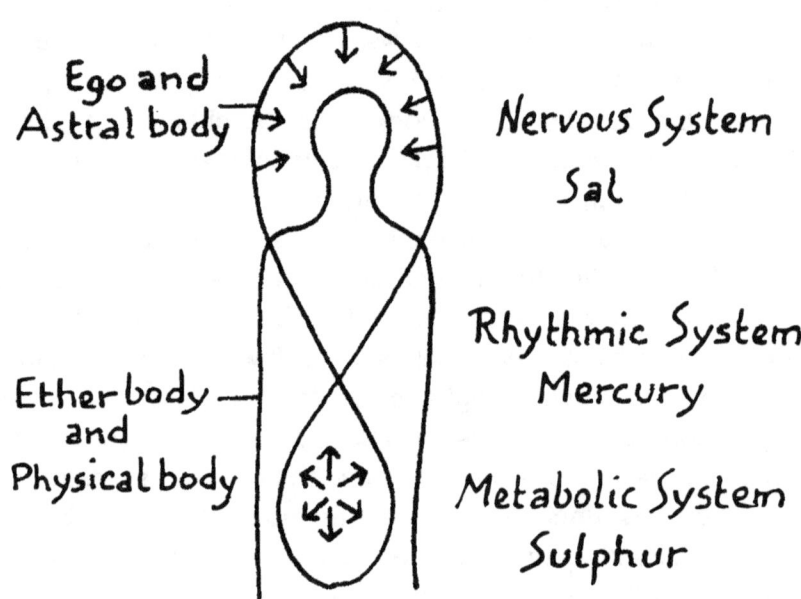

Let us note at the outset that the two lower members, physical body and ether body, form a stronger connection with each other, as opposed to astral body and ego which again are more closely connected. This is demonstrated by the fact that in sleep astral body and ego leave the nerve-sense domain and return again on awakening. In the night, the nerve organs are flooded by upbuilding processes and restored. Waking and sleeping is a rhythmical function and its disturbances, which may have the most varied causes, are influenced most beneficially by Rhythmical Massage.

In the drawing, astral body and ego are symbolized through a lemniscate because these two members insert themselves into the general organism via the system of breathing. As a consequence of the fact that we are bearers of a soul, the bodily organization must be imprinted with the polarity between nerve system and metabolic system. The animal and human bodies first show this in contrast to the plants which only need the insertion of an ether body. In the picture language of the Bible this process of ensouling is described—as we have already stated—with the words: 'And God breathed into his nostrils the breath of life.' There arises an indentation, the astral body invaginates the plant principle, all the glands including the lungs are invaginated trees, the lungs are the center of the invaginated air organism. The plant is still breathed at from outside, it is embedded in the macrocosmic air organism of the earth. We can follow up the ranks of animals and see how the breathing process of the skin in the lowest animals gradually draws more and more inward until it ends in the formation of the lungs. Because of this movement toward the inside which is connected with the insertion of soul and spirit we have to represent its function by a lemniscate which as a curve shows this breathing oscillation. There arise, quite distinctly, two domains, an upper and a lower one. Above, the astral body acts from outside, shaping and breaking down, upon the physical and etheric bodies via the nerve-sense system which it had left after having built up this instrument in the unconscious embryonic period. Below, the astral body plunges deep down into the metabolic processes and gives the impulses to act from inside outward. This submersion is the basis for growth, nutrition, and so on, but never for consciousness. In the embryo and in early childhood the upbuilding processes predominate. During this period the astral body fashions its instrument in order later to free itself of it and to use it from outside. That means: the astral body builds up in this period the marvellous structure of the nervous system like a congealed mirror image of itself, in order to use this mirror for the formation of thoughts by again breaking it down.

The lemniscate clearly shows this polaric connection of functions. The crossing point conceived as a picture of motion corresponds to the rhythmical processes of inhalation and exhalation which bring about the transition and equilibrium. From this it follows that the higher members of man's being take hold of the body through a rhythmical process of which we are not entirely conscious. In every movement of will the path leads from visualization through a rhythmical process to will-forming metabolic processes.

That is the reason why all disturbances in the field of movement may be relieved and improved through Rhythmical Massage.

If we closely observe this relatively simple diagram which only shows the fundamental laws, we shall immediately understand the concepts *Sal, Sulphur,* and *Mercury* which Paracelsus introduced into medicine, basing them on alchemistic traditions. Paracelsus still had the possibility of beholding the ether body which he called 'Archaeus.' In the three names *Sal, Sulphur,* and *Mercury,* are concealed the three spheres of function of the nerve-sense system, the rhythmical processes, and metabolism.

Salt formation (*Sal*) is a process through which from living fluid dead matter is excreted. At the basis of every process of consciousness there lies a delicate salt formation (not measurable with coarse instruments); that is, a weakened death process, a mineralization process. The imponderables withdraw from the *Sal* and surround it. *Sal* formation is simultaneously a materialization process from a finer to a denser medium.

Sulphur is the polar opposite; all metabolic processes are sulphuric, *Sulphur* absorbs the imponderable. Substance is dissolved from inside outward; it is rarefied and can be smelled. It has a relationship to warmth. *Sal*, on the other hand, is cold.

If we compare these processes with those in the plant, the blossom process is to be called sulphuric, it is a dematerialization process. The root process is of the nature of *Sal*; here matter is stored in lasting forms.

If we compare man and plant, it becomes evident that the plant is present in man in reverse order (see R. Hauschka, *Nutrition*).*

The health-supporting rhythmical processes of the middle system are called *Mercury* by Paracelsus, represented in the Mercury staff with the lemniscate of the two snakes which are to be thought of in swinging motion. Mercury was able to bind and to release, to put to sleep and to awaken. What was it he could bind and release? The spirit-soul element, the astral body, carrying the ego, he was able to release into sleep and to bind into awakening. The images of mythology are quite exact if we are willing to enter into them.

If we have a correct conception of these great functional laws of the ether body, that is to say, of the physiological plane of events in man, we can go very far in assessing a curative measure such as massage. Since the days of Hippocrates, as reported in the chapter 'The History of Massage,' massage consists in the final analysis in a *differentiated binding and releasing*, in the possibility on the one hand of strengthening the connection of the members of man's being through rhythmical motion, of bringing about a deeper immersion of spirit and soul into the body or, on the other hand, of releasing them from the body in order to restore the generally or locally disturbed equilibrium.

Since the etheric body is the architect of the physical body, it must first be grasped in its threefold web of laws. The fourfold physical body, the earthly, the fluid, the aeriform, and the warmth body, all take part in the threefold membering, for the ether body permeates the whole physical body. In the following descriptions of the water organism, the air and warmth organisms, it will be shown in how far the polarity of the

---

*   Rudolf Steiner Press, London 1979.

Sal and *Sulphur* processes and the *Mercury* principle of the middle appear ever and again as the regulating functional threefold membering.

A description of the solid organism, of anatomy, is presupposed, and will not be considered here.

4.

THE WATER ORGANISM

It is always difficult to describe the water, air, and warmth organisms singly, for they are all interconnected and permeate one another. Just as the elements of nature intermingle, so do the higher entities, life, soul and spirit working in them, interact. Yet each single one is an organism.

The fluid element, water, bringing the celestial forces to the earth, was revered in all the ancient cultures as a holy element. Man always turned to water when he sought healing from too great an entanglement with the earth sphere. The dust of the earth was washed off his feet. Near a well one felt the nearness of the heavens, for cosmic wisdom lived in its domain. Odin drew it from Mimir's well. Divine powers, so men thought, reach down into the life-bestowing fluid element. Every sanctuary had its well. To sit beside flowing waters permeates the human soul with an inkling of the transitoriness of the earthly; selfless renunciation takes hold of the soul and longing for its heavenly home touches it. The water beings in all fairy tales and sagas are full of longing, and they strive up into the lighter air element.

The waters of the earth, like the air, are an interconnected organism that guarantees the life of the globe. We are beginning to realize how true this is, since our technology spreads so much death. The qualities of water, the fluid element, are shaped through the *laws of the etheric world*. Therefore the three processes *Sal*, *Sulphur*, and *Mercury*, that is to say salt formation and structuring, loosening transformation, and rhythmical balance, are present in water. It does not have its individual form, but complies with any form; it repeats on earth the cosmic sphere. If the surface differences were equalized, the earth would have a water mantle of a depth of one and a half kilometers. The *cosmic world of forces*, warmth, light, chemical forces, and life, permeate everywhere the water organism of the earth. It pulsates in the tides according to cosmic rhythms, warm and cold currents flow through it. Water as element is able to dissolve the salt of the earth, to absorb the higher forces of light and warmth and rhythmically to mingle with the air. The fluid element is thus the mediator between the salt-forming, contracting earth forces and the dissolving forces of light and warmth. The forming principle also shows itself in the skin formation of the surface which creates a tension, enabling small insects to walk over it. It shows itself, on the other hand, in the dissolving principle through the immense power of digestion of the oceans and rivers, and, finally, in the rhythmical principle of rising and falling, of evaporation and condensation, in high tide and low tide. The meandering of rivers also shows a rhythmical character. Indeed, in every living cell there pulses the liquid protoplasm. Theodor Schwenk's book *Sensitive Chaos** gives deep insight into the nature of water.

The sum total of these qualities makes the element water the ideal sphere of all life processes. In former times the entire field of medicine was directed toward the fluid element in man; its quality, the good or bad mixture of the fluids, decided between health and sickness.

Up to the beginning of our natural-scientific age all therapy was based on observation of the fluid in man.

The water organism of man is an enlivened unit, although in it countless individual currents swing together. It shows an organization which corresponds to the functional threefold membering of the human organism. *The metabolic fluids* are living, sulphuric, turbid; within them and in the fluid cell content of the metabolic organs there take place the innumerable combinations and transformations of matter which belong to organic life. These processes end in the preparation of blood. Blood and its circulation are the middle part of the water organism. Through the impulse of breathing it acquires a definite rhythm. This circulation is not merely a circulation in the ordinary sense; the blood is radiated from its center in the heart, is thrown to the periphery as a whole and in every organ in particular and is again absorbed in the heart. This is a movement which could never be carried out by a pump. To the heart a much higher significance is due. We have seen that the astral body with its relationship to the forces of the stars enters circulation through breathing; it gives impulses to the ether body from inside. In us there is a force, resembling the movement of the stars, which the astral body imprints upon the ether body and which takes the blood along, just as outside, the starry rhythms, imprinted in the ether body of the earth, cause the tides and the rising and falling of the saps in the plants. The ether body is in continuous motion. Only in the physical body matters are fixed, resting in space. In the ether or life body which permeates the water organism, everything is in motion. Transforming and interweaving rhythms caused in it by the astral body flow in it. When it stands still it is in the process of dying.

The part of the water organism which only slightly circulates belongs to the death processes of the head. It must not contain anything but a trace of salt in order not to disturb through too much life the process of consciousness which needs the *Sal* state of the fluid. The *cerebrospinal fluid* and the *fluids of the sense organs* are places from which life has almost completely withdrawn. That is to say, the ether body has partially lifted itself out in order to serve the consciousness process. The lifted-out part of our

---

*   Rudolf Steiner Press, London, 1965.

ether body is the basis for our life of thought and perception, for our forces of fantasy, for the 'fluidic' course of our thought processes.

We think according to the same laws that are to be found in growth. Readiness for school in the child is reached when the organs have been developed, the ether forces freeing themselves more and more in order to become the basis of his conscious soul life. If we demand too early achievements of the child in the intellectual sphere, we have to expect defectively developed organs and, later on, serious damage. If the ether body liberates itself from the water organism, devitalizing processes appear; if it unites itself more closely with the body of fluids, more intensive life is stimulated. Thus there exist in the man of fluids various *stages of vitality*. Three realms come into being: First, the reproductive and metabolic fluids which are turbid and rich in cells, but very vital; second, the blood which passes through rhythmically changing states of enhanced life and mildly destructive processes in the red and blue blood; and, finally, the clear fluids of the sense-nerve system which are almost mineralized. A sketch may illustrate this.

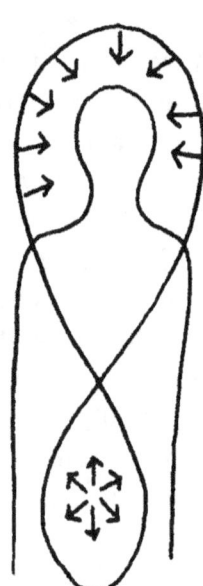

Nerve System
Cerebro-spinal fluid

Rhythmic System
Arterial and Venous blood

Metabolic System
Chyle and Lymph

Levity rules in the entire water organism. This has a special significance in the head although the principle holds good for all solid deposits. The floating brain is lifted out of gravity to enable us to think. For it presses upon its vascular basis with the weight of only 20 grams. Thought function needs the resting mirror. In the heart-lung system, however, the water organism receives the impulses of the sun rhythm of breath and pulse frequency. This will be explained in the chapter 'Circulation and Heart.' There is never rest, which would signify death, but rhythmical motion predominates. In the metabolic sphere, that is to say, in the life functions, the organism of fluids is directed by the liver. It is the mysterious alchemistic laboratory of our transformation of matter. It receives the entire fluid of nutrition from the intestinal region through the portal vein which nourishes the liver. Here the most varied life processes take hold of substance. The cosmic rhythm gives way to individual, arbitrary impulses of motion, and the main stress lies on the continuous chemical-alchemical transformations of substances.

For Rhythmical Massage it is important to pay heed to this water organism through the quality of the grip. All pulsating, streaming grips are able to serve the vitalizing of the tissues, all sucking grips serve the forces of levity and reabsorption, all modelling grips serve the shaping and solidification of the ether body in the physical body.

We shall deal with this in detail later on. Here we have endeavored to awaken a new consciousness, a sensitive comprehension for this life-endowed fluid human being.

5.

THE AIR ORGANISM

The air organism, too, is a totality, although it is hardly possible to draw it. It is closely connected with the water organism since the air or gaseous element dips down into the blood in breathing. Half of the air organism is immersed in water. If, however, the astral body, controlling it, does not dip down properly, there appear in the metabolic realm separate air bodies causing flatulence. In the metabolic system air ought to be dissolved in the fluids.

Much can be gained for the observation of the air organism if we acquire a sensitive understanding of the nature of air through the observation of the phenomena in the atmosphere of the earth.—I point once more to the excellent book by Theodor Schwenk: *Sensitive Chaos.*—The air sheath of the earth, too, is a totality. The air movements in it take place between the polarity of high pressure and low pressure areas. Immense air bodies move between pole and equator. The phenomena change rapidly, and meteorological maps have to be drawn anew daily. Certain storms have a definite character and it is out of a deep instinct that hurricanes are given names, even today. All conditions change in the air element much more quickly, we might even say, capriciously, than in water. In the above mentioned book the air movements, the sensitive, *irritable character* of the air is presented in many examples, scientifically and also imaginatively. The author emphasizes how everything takes place faster, more acutely, more quiveringly. The wind rises and is gone, a sudden squall races over the water, building up enormous waves in no time. Another special quality of air is its elasticity. Water cannot be compressed but air can, whereby its inner tension increases as it condenses, and the pressure may be discharged in explosion.

Such drastic examples show us that the air or the gaseous element is shaped by the soul-astral forces. It is impossible to give here an exhaustive description of the connection of the element air with the astral realm that permeates it.

The astral, the soul, bestows *consciousness* and *motion* upon man; it is an inwardness related to light; it is inexhaustibly deep like the stellar spaces. We have little knowledge of the atmosphere since we observe it merely physically; it is interwoven with *states of light* as is our soul with states of consciousness; it is also interwoven with the *formative forces* that radiate down from the starry cosmos. Effects are radiated down from sun and moon and all the planets. The atmosphere is the mediator of all this. Its miracles of color and sound are eternally changing, like our feelings, and bear witness to the fact that it, too, represents an inwardness and is a mirror of a world soul being. The Egyptians still perceived in the morning and evening glow manifestations of the world soul. They called it 'Isis.' Isis was the celestial all. They looked up to the celestial-all perceiving in it the creator powers of the organs of the physical body. Isis, the world soul, created the organ of the ensouling of man, the lungs. Osiris, the sun power, made the breath creative in speech and created the larynx. Both together—so it was imagined—created Horus, the heart, in the motherly embrace of the lungs.

Let us return to our microcosmic air organism. All soul stirrings immediately affect breathing, as everyone can observe. Thus the air organism leads into the body all the forces of our individual astral body; through it the *impulses* penetrate right into the physical body. The Greeks still possessed a sure feeling for this. When they walked, they said: 'Mars gives me the impulse for it;' when they lay down, it was Saturn that surrendered them to gravity; when they sat, they felt in themselves the throning power of Jupiter. They still knew that all the impulses to inner activity originated in the astral body, the celestial soul of man which carries the Ego. This fact, extended into a cosmic image, was seen in Isis with her son Horus.

There is a phenomenon that shows the connection between the processes in the air organism of the earth and those in the microcosm man, the connection that the Egyptians would have described as that between the world soul and the human soul. If the air organism of man has not become sufficiently independent of the outer world, it reacts morbidly to the movements of the atmosphere. This is especially the case if through cyclones cold air moves in below warm air, enclosing it. A so-called occlusion results. Even before instruments indicate any changes in air pressure, it may trigger fits of choking, strokes, pneumonia and hemorrhages. These, of course, are extreme cases, but everyone knows the pains in old scars and all kinds of indispositions caused by changes in the weather.

In the air organism, too, we can distinguish three domains that have the character of *Sal*, *Mercury*, and *Sulphur*.

In the *head region* the *air spaces* are *stationary*, the air apparently being exchanged very slowly; for instance, in the sinuses of the head bones.

In the *rhythmic system* we have the *function of breathing*, the actual *great Mercury process*, in which are concealed all the secrets of healing if only it is followed through right into its finest ramifications and effects in the organism. For breathing and circulation are the great equalization systems between the two poles of the nerve and metabolic processes which, if left to themselves, would cause illnesses. Here binding and loosening, the deep penetration and again releasing of the spirit-soul element, has been raised to a rhythmical function. We might say that here is intertwined the great rhythm of incarnation and excarnation, earthly life and resurrection in the spirit. Birth and death, sleeping and waking, inhalation and exhalation are the great *Mercury* functions that were symbolized in earlier ages through the staff of serpents which Apollo bestowed upon Mercury. A deeper consideration will discover that these functions are three great blessings that signify healing for the maladies of human existence.

The transformation of substances takes place in the *sulphur sphere of metabolism*. Here the sulphurizing flame burns which leads the substances back out of the earth element into the higher elements, right up into warmth, heat. This is a dematerializing process, a *dissolving* process, in which the submerged part of the air organism takes part.

Just as the *water organism* has its special relationship to the *liver*, so the *air organism* is connected with the *kidney*. It is the kidney that needs most oxygen and produces the strong desire for air. It irradiates our air organism with inner states of light. In the chapter about the inner cosmic system of our organs, the function of the kidney will be dealt with in detail.

Through the air organism we *ensoul* the whole body. During the embryonic state the soul or the astral body still works from outside, shaping the sheaths of the embryo. Later with the first breath and the development of the lungs we draw it more deeply inwards. Then only are we incarnated properly. The word 'caro' means flesh. Breathing maintains throughout life the connection of spirit and soul with the body. When breathing ceases, life dies.

For massage it is important to enter with one's feeling into the bodily activity of the astral. The astral body branches from the breathing center into the polarity of the *forming of consciousness* and *movement*. These are the two qualities that raise us above the plant, which has no soul. The astral body imprints its character upon the air organism and is placed above the ether body. From above it imprints form upon it and from inside, immersed into it, it gives it impetus. The air is permeated by formative forces. This can be seen in the formation of clouds. Schwenk speaks of differentiated air bodies having sensitive surfaces.

If one is able to introduce this intimate knowledge into the movements of massage, the astral body will be especially engaged. The impulses in the quality of the grip, the differentiated shaping, producing consciousness, attracts the astral body. Not a dreamlike spread-out motion, but the consciously localized work wakes up the astral body. This astral body concerns us as the pacemaker of the ego if we wish to learn in a new way the meaning of binding and releasing in the sense of Hippocrates. In the present book only the first characteristics can be given, the direction can be indicated in which an understanding of the new method of massage can be looked for. Knowledge of man can only slowly be acquired. The microcosm man is anything but a technically surveyable factory or mechanism for which parts are readily available or which may be repaired according to mechanical laws. It is an infinitely complicated interplay of celestial and terrestrial forces, of the soul-spiritual and the physical-bodily. Rudolf Steiner's Science of the Spirit offers concepts that enable us slowly to penetrate with our knowledge into this microcosm.

6.

THE WARMTH ORGANISM

After having advanced from the purely physical earth body, which belongs to the mineral world, to the observation of the water organism, which carries life because it is permeated by the etheric body, and having further advanced to the observation of the air organism, which with its inner light conditions carries the soul, we now have to observe the warmth organism that makes us a bearer of the spirit.

The first human being who received a philosophical instruction about these relationships was the young Alexander the Great, who was initiated by Aristotle into his teaching of the elements. Much that is found in the activities of the alchemists can be traced back to him.

A diagram will make this clear.

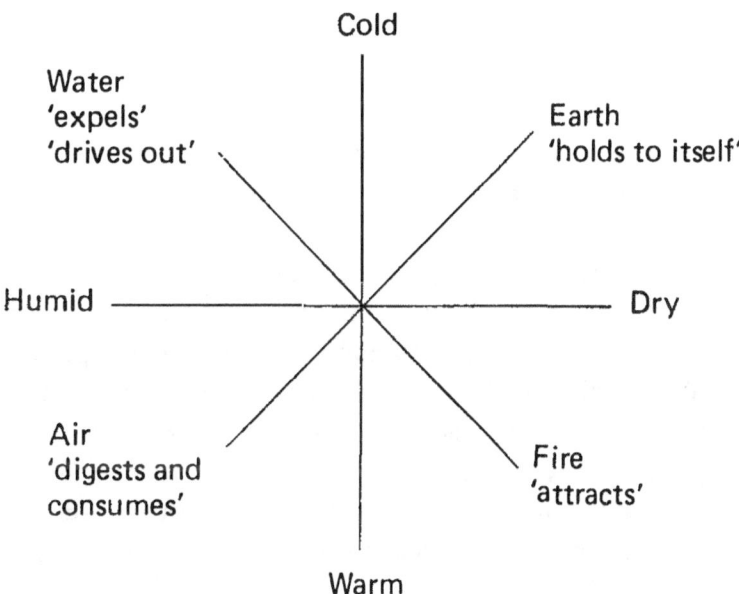

In olden times one proceeded always from experiences, and the qualities cold, warm, dry, humid constitute the starting point. The elements themselves form a second cross, their qualities intersecting. The element earth is cold and dry, water is cold and humid; and so on. Added to this, the utterances of the alchemists, which have come down to us from the time of Paracelsus and even earlier, are distinct indications of the relationship of the elements to the higher members of man's being. The earth 'holds to itself,' encloses itself, solidifies. The water 'expels;' that is to say, the plant that has only an etheric body, only vegetative life, drives out the higher members, fights against their penetration. The air 'digests and consumes;' the soul element that is added in the animals, instinct, desires, passions, they 'feed' upon the juices of life, they break down substances. The fire 'attracts;' it draws the spirit into itself as the magnet does the iron. On the paths of warmth the spiritual works right down into the physical.

Warmth is the bridge between the sensory and the supersensory world; it stands on the boundary between material and spiritual world; today we no longer consider it as an actual element into which every substance may be raised.

In the evolutionary doctrine of the Science of the Spirit warmth stands at the beginning of creation. Spiritual warmth, *divine fire of creation*, gradually condenses in physically measurable warmth. Through enthusiasm we can still today warm ourselves physically, and in reverse, physical warmth produced by the metabolic processes can be changed into spirit-soul warmth. We do not live in order to eat, but in order to develop heat warmth for the spirit wishing to reveal itself creatively upon the earth.

Thus the warmth organism is of a significance that is tremendous, though not easily assessed. Fire stands not only at the beginning of evolution. It stands, in the narrower sense, at the beginning of culture, because culture signifies the impulse of the spirit in the life of nations. Thus I should like to call fire a *hierarchical substance*, the effluence of the divine creator hierarchies. Warmth is never a 'by-product,' but presupposition for all spiritual and bodily activity of the human spirit. This is a short circumscription of the fact that our individuality, the I, governs all other functions, through the *independent warmth organism*, activating, comprising and leading them to the essentially human. We carry within us mineral, plant, and animal processes but all of them have finally to be raised to the human stage through the presence of the ego in the warmth organism. This already starts in the development of the embryo. In the animal experiment an interruption of the brood warmth is of catastrophic consequences for bodily development. Stump formation of the limbs and an ectopic heart (i.e., transposition toward the outside) have been observed. This throws a light upon the fact that the warmth organism is particularly *anchored in the heart*. The heart, our inner sun, is the physical center of our spiritual existence. The brain, in contrast, is only the intelligent mirror, the cerebral life is a changeful life in pictures. We think this, and tomorrow that. The world of thought, of visualizations, is a world of reflections. The feeling of existence, however, is bound up more with the life of the heart. Here, there lives conscience, the sense of responsibility, loyalty, and similar qualities bound up with the core of the individuality.

Let us sketch the warmth organism. It, too, has two distinct poles, but it unites them into a complete unity. Since it is chiefly anchored in the blood, it is strongly connected in the lower man with the metabolic organs. Here physical warmth is produced; special sources of warmth development are liver activity, kidney activity, and movement of the muscles.

In the upper man, the warmth organism envelops the nerve system, it strives toward the outside and much warmth is lost. Many people sitting in a hall heat the space through these radiations of the upper warmth organism, and not with their feet, though exhalation also contributes. The warmth organism is especially active wherever the ego has shaped and works in the body; that is, in the heart, the hands and the face. In blushing and in growing pale we can observe the flooding up and down of the waves of warmth.

It is well known that the temperature of the feet rises in sleep and in anaesthesia. If the ego in sleep, carried by the astral body, is lifted out of the nerve-sense man, it unites more deeply with metabolic man. Then the body must be protected against excessive cooling off. Also in states of exhaustion man needs a greater supply of warmth from outside. Especially in accidents with loss of consciousness care has to be taken that the person in question does not cool off too much. In the morning, man takes hold of his body starting in the feet. We could visualize this process in a kind of circulatory movement. Ego and astral body release themselves in sleep from the nerve-sense system and take hold of the body in the morning through the will organism.

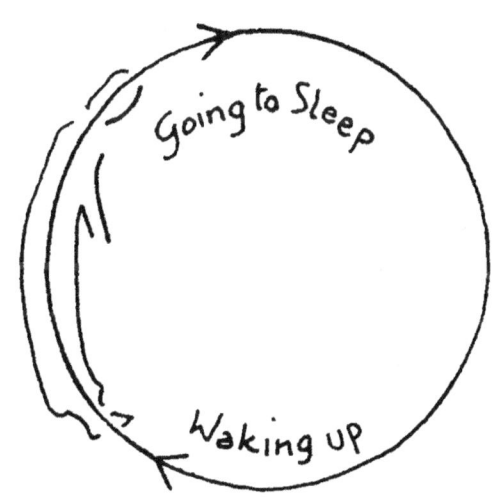

Circulatory Movement of the Ego and Astral Body in Sleep

The ego giving structure to the warmth organism can maintain itself at an outside temperature between +60° and -60° C. Naturally, the boundaries cannot be determined with accuracy. With inside temperatures the difference is much smaller and amounts to but a few degrees.

By sub-temperature, all the processes are slowed down, by increase of warmth they are accelerated and activated. If we are 'freezing cold' or only 'shivering', the warmth organism contracts, as is the case at the beginning of an acute state of fever. It begins with damming up of warmth toward the inside, a violent push of the ego into the body. Only then the warmth organism expands again in fever.

Since warmth is the body of the ego, paths of warmth are needed in order to enable the ego to appear everywhere in the organism as giver of equilibrium, as highest resource for the humanization of all processes. If this is not possible, it signifies the beginning of many diseases.

Therefore, the whole human being is employed in the regulation of warmth, in the metabolic system through changes of the production of warmth, in the rhythmical system through expansion and contraction of the capillaries as well as through changes in the breathing frequency and, finally, in the skin, belonging to the nerve-sense system, through secretion of perspiration as a breaking down and cooling process.

Motility in connection with the problem of warmth will be dealt with in the chapter, 'The Muscle System.'

Finally, let us return to the idea of warmth forming the bridge between body and spirit, which is possible through the fact that physical warmth can be transmuted into etheric warmth.

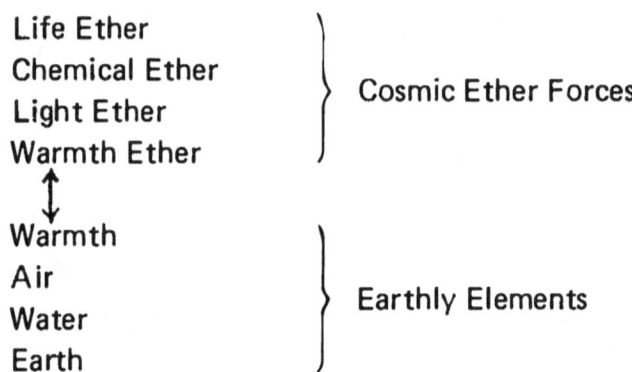

Physical warmth is the uppermost of the earthly elements, warmth ether is the lowest of the etheric formative forces. The elements, as well as the formative forces active in them, have arisen in world evolution one after the other. In his book *Occult Science—An Outline*, Rudolf Steiner shows through the three pre-states of the earth the slow development of primeval fire into ever higher ether forces on the one hand, and, on the other into the accompanying states of condensation, until finally on the earth the element 'Earth' or the mineral, dead element arises and, above, the life ether, the formative force, that endows the formed bodies with earthly life. The following drawing may clarify this.

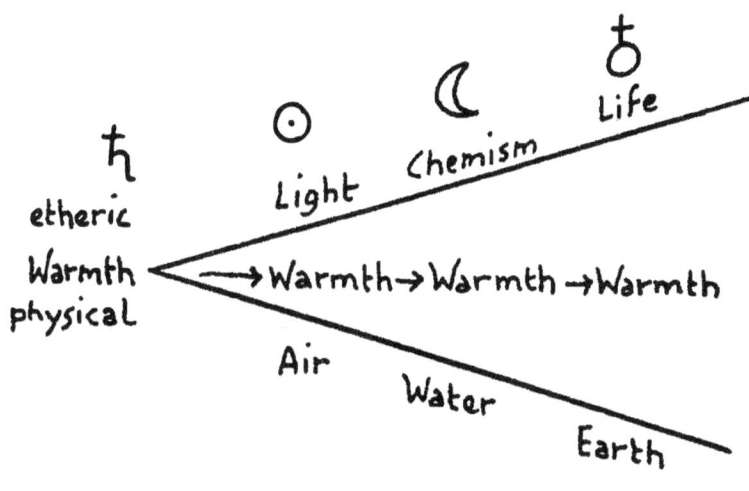

World Evolution and the Elements

These facts demonstrate the central position of the element fire through all the planetary pre-states which are repeated by the earth at the beginning of its evolution.

When these formative forces are connected with the world of substances of our physical body and call it into 'life,' earthly life results. The spiritual life of man has as its basis the free ether forces that are carried, held together, and enclosed by fire.

In the warmth organism of our head there takes place a continual alternation of physical activity and spiritual activity. If the physical warmth is the basis for the bodily activity of the ego, the etheric warmth that streams to the head is the basis for our ego-permeated space of consciousness.

At the beginning of every culture there is the master of fire, but without the etherized fire, without the warmth ether, there is no spiritual culture, no life of knowledge.

Our turning to the world with interest is already a walking on paths of warmth. Wonder, astonishment, which are the beginning of all wisdom, are in themselves a gentle warming of the soul. Wherever our spirit turns, it can only move on the stages of warmth development, the unfolding of warmth in the physical, etheric and soul realms. If warmth is lacking as a basis, everything falls asunder. If our thinking becomes ''cold' we have, as Goethe says, only 'the parts in our hand.' The great inter-relationships that characterize the far-seeing spirit are lost. This process of transition from physical to to etheric warmth, this etherization of the blood, in Rudolf Steiner's designation, is the uppermost level of our physical processes; here everything flows into the spiritual. If the flame of spiritualized blood warmth is burning in us in the vessel of the head, as it were, we are able, through special intensification of our life of knowledge, to come into contact with the objective world of spirit.

Warmth as element carries the whole Christian development of the ego, the I. This radiates through Christian Morgenstern's line: 'To Thee I lift my heart as a genuine vessel of the Grail,' into which the Holy Spirit in the shape of a dove lets flow healing celestial forces. For the imaginative pictures of the history of the Grail are concerned with the secrets of the connection of Blood, Ego, and World-Spirit. They describe the path upon which the human spirit finds the cosmic spirit.

There should no longer be any doubt about the fact that care for the warmth organism is the supreme law and task of medicine founded on the spirit.

It may be fostered and stimulated from the bodily as well as the spiritual aspect. Our culture is no longer conscious of its fundamental significance. We live in a constant battle for the foundations of the human spirit and create, through its denial, a host of diseases caused by cold, and also physical as well as spiritual phenomena of decay.

The wise men of the Middle Ages knew how to value fire in its all-pervading significance; this is shown by an old fire verse of the Rosicrucians. In it, a fourfold fire was indicated which was witness to the fact that there still existed remnants of ancient knowledge that reflected the old wisdom of the elements concerning the four formative forces that correspond to four states of world evolution.

A similar echo may be found with Paracelsus in his designation of the mixture of fluids underlying the four temperaments.

The fire verse:

> Strive for the fire, seek for the fire,
> Thou shalt become fire.
> Bring fire to fire, broil fire in fire,
> Throw body, soul and spirit into fire,
> Then hast thou dead and living fire,
> Thou shalt become black, yellow, white, red fire.
> Bear thy children in fire,
> Give them food and drink in fire,
> Thus they live and die in fire,
> And are and will remain in fire,
> Their silver and gold shall all become fire
> And shall be in the end a fourfold philosophic fire.

7.

NERVE AND BLOOD

Using the example of nerve and blood I shall once more describe the polarity of the upper and lower parts of man. I am fully conscious of the fact that, in separating the physiological process into its basic tendencies, we must not forget that the threefold membering is not a threefold partitioning. In reality, three whole human beings are inserted into one another, the nerve-sensory man, the rhythmical man and the metabolic man. Difficulties arise through the fact that the great laws repeat themselves in every detail. Man is a microcosm. It is not to be expected that he can be quickly and simply understood or adequately described. But a start has to be made. For every human being, even though he has no medical training, should have a general comprehension of the great processes of his body, of illness and health, quite especially those who work in curative establishments as assistants of the physician.

In this book, therefore, the subjects are described to the extent in which they relate to the comprehension of massage.

Let us consider once more the two polar spheres: the nerve system and, as exponent of the metabolic system, the blood. The nerve system has the character of Sal, as we have seen. It is a secretion of the whole life process; in other words, it no longer contains much of the forces of reproduction, to some extent even none at all, making destruction in it final. When it has developed, spirit (ego) and soul (astral body) withdraw from it, organizing it no longer or only slightly from inside; they use it from outside. Even the etheric body partially withdraws in order to become the basis for the processes of consciousness. The nerve system, having little life itself, must be kept alive by the blood flowing around it, thus receiving life from the metabolic system, preventing it from complete death in us. Our conscious life causes a constant slow *decay of nerve substance*. At the price of a death process slowly poisoning us, we are able to gain on earth awareness and consciousness of self. The wondrous structure of our brain, the indescribably differentiated web of our nervous system, is an image, congealed into form, of our astral body, an image of the starry world, of our starlight nature. It is the archetypal image. The whole nervous system is *permeated by a web of cosmic laws*. We have twelve senses, twelve doors to the universe; as the sun moves through the twelve signs of the zodiac, so our spirit moves through twelve spheres of the senses. The spinal cord with its twenty-eight to thirty-one segments is determined by the rhythm of the moon of twenty-eight to thirty-one days. The sympathetic nervous system, immersed into the metabolic region of the lower man, has remained more alive. It, therefore, does not mediate consciousness and has like lower plants the texture of vegetative formations. The central nervous system has the structure of fibres originating from light structures, light paths in the astral body that have gradually condensed into the forms of the nervous system. The brain that comprises all these radiations may be considered a kind of concave mirror. For the nervous system acts only centripetally, it is no telephone station, as many people would like to believe, into which one can speak commands, in order for example to summon a muscle to move. No, it is only the *total instrument of perception* for our ego, enabling us to survey the entire extent of our microcosm. This is of especial importance if we wish to conceive how movements come into existence. The motor nervous system tells us the location of the muscle we wish to move. Anything with which I am not connected by a nerve is outer world for my ego. It is beyond my control and becomes as foreign to me as any other object outside. The path from thought to execution of a movement passes always through a rhythmical process into the metabolism which must form the basis for the unfolding of will through a warmth process. These relationships will be dealt with more explicitly in regard to paralysis in the chapter, 'The Muscle System.'

Thus, the nervous system and its functions are directed from the outside inwards. Every stimulus runs from the sense sphere toward the center up to the brain that is that wondrous mirror which enables us to reproduce the entire universe, not physically, to be sure, but spiritually. The force of reproduction of the ether body has freed itself from the body and has turned toward the soul. In other words, *the forces of growth of the ether body transform themselves in the course of evolution into forces of thinking*. The more the body is developed the more do ether forces become free and serve the soul for its processes of consciousness. This holds good for the development of school maturity right up to the wisdom of old age. In our time this connection is not realized. People would like to remain physically young and capable of reproduction, yet they pay for this with a certain lack of the wisdom of old age.

The behavior of blood with its sulphuric character is the polar opposite of what has been described above. It has little permanency and dies at once if it is no longer contained within the form of the body. Blood is a creation of the earth, it is formed in the embryo on the yolk, the first earthly nutriment, whereas the inception of the nervous system is an indentation from outside, out of the amniotic sac. The first inception of the spinal cord is a dorsal furrow. From the very beginning, astral body and ego connect themselves more strongly with the blood. When the blood of the mother has ended its period of activity, they immerse themselves with the first breath more deeply into the blood of the child and from there into the body. This is the actual incarnation which decides about the fundamental connection of the soul-spiritual with the body. From this moment the blood of the child plays the role of the constant source of renewal. On the other hand, the metabolism ends in the blood. The level of blood processes is, as it were, the highest level of metabolism where it already takes part in rhythm. As differentiated as is the nerve-sense system, so the blood streams uniformly through our vessels. It has the impulse to move into the periphery and is sucked back through the sucking power of the ether body. The astral body immersed into the blood brings forth the pulse, produces the tone everywhere that works from inside outward; it is a radiating, centrifugal process in contrast to the raying in, the centripetal direction of the nerve-sense process. Wherever the blood arrives it brings along the force of regeneration. Wounds do not heal without intensive blood activity. Blood and nerve, which exist in mutual biological tension as the one entices the other into action until an equilibrium is achieved, always act together. One may compare their mutual relationship with that of positive and negative electricity. The balance is attained by the rhythmical activities of the middle man.

Whereas from above there stream downward the formative and secretory forces out of the domain of the nerve-sense system, there flows upward the living stream of nutrition and growth. A wound forms granulations out of the blood forces, but the proper formation of tissue into the human shape derives from the forces mediated by the nervous system. If the lower stream overpowers growth, so-called 'wild flesh' is formed, and so forth. Blood and nerve confront one another like two systems, the one of which secretes sediments out of the fluid, introducing a condensation process, a mineralization process, whereas the other system is able to dissolve these sediments, indeed, sulphurizing them into spiritualization. This means the blood is able to activate a dematerializing process. Human blood is a substance, as Rudolf Steiner describes it, that continually dissolves into etheric substance, it 'vaporizes', we might say. Thus, in the human being these two poles interact continuously and everywhere, but in the whole household of life the condensations and excretions must have a certain relationship to the processes of growth and dissolution; only then are we healthy from inside. Both poles in their onesidedness would make us ill. We see clearly that health is the individual balance of the processes which must in every human being be produced through his rhythmical processes.

The great polar processes of metabolic activity in the blood and nerve-sense activity must exist in their onesidedness in order that man may manifest consciousness and motion, although each by itself may lead to illness. To become acquainted with them in their origin and anatomy as well as in the way of their activity is of great importance because the rhythmical movements in the middle man, connected with systole and diastole, are the health-giving forms of motion that can especially in massage be used in great differentiation. Systole and diastole are essential in breath as well as in pulse. Formative contraction and loosening suction are qualities of manipulation that imitate exactly the activity of the rhythmical system. Hippocrates was right when he said that everything rests on binding and loosening. We shall have to describe the hand as predestined tool for the activation of these two qualities harmoniously united.

8.

CIRCULATION AND HEART

In massage, special attention is paid to circulation and heart. They are the central happening in the organism of fluids in man, indeed, in the human body in general. From the side of metabolism, all building-up processes flow into the circulating blood; so do, from the other side, all breaking down processes accompanying the conscious activity of the nerve-sense system. Thus blood is the place where all life processes meet and unite, where in the stream of time life flows on in eternal metamorphoses. The physiological, chemical processes that accompany all functions taking their course in time culminate in the blood. Here they are collected by the ego of man, perceived in their quality and harmonized as far as possible. 'Who can say that he understands the blood!' says Novalis. This is a fully justified utterance, for the blood, this 'special juice' can only be described from quite definite aspects. For only if a person were to have advanced to the ultimate mysteries of the individuality, of the human spirit, could he understand the warm blood formed by this spirit and following its impulses. The blood is the most mobile and most readily influenced of our system of organs. The same holds good of the heart which becomes the center of circulation from the moment when with the first breath the spirit and soul of man enter the body that they have built up during embryonic development. In fetal and embryonic circulation matters are different. Only in the third stage, the development of the circulation of the born human being through the closing of the separating heart wall, the heart gains its final central position.

If one considers circulation from the standpoint of the members of man's being, the purely natural-scientific conceptions of today must be modified. The ether body permeating the fluid man with forces and deriving its impulses from the higher members of man's being is *the mover of the blood*. Circulation already begins outside the embryo at the wall of the yolk sac; cells are loosened and stream in developing capillaries growing into the embryo. Also inside the embryo the capillaries begin to grow, everything unites later in the third week. The blood flows before the heart exists. To be sure, the heart begins to take shape earlier but is completed only in the third month. Also later on *the heart never acts as a pump*. It is the organ which *produces the rhythm of the blood stream*. Rudolf Steiner would allow the heart to be compared with a ram, but never with a pump. In every systole the heart motion separates the stream into a sequence of large drops, it interrupts the stream up to a momentary standstill only at once to release the blood again. This rhythm provides us with the feeling of time, we experience dimly our rhythm of life. A uniform circulation would not be able to provide us with a consciousness of time. We usually speak of circulation in observing the blood motion and imagine a kind of circle. Besides this, however, the blood motion is a dispersion into the periphery and a sucking back, and this gesture is repeated in every single organ. Seen as a whole the blood is dispersed three times, upward, downward, and into the two lungs. In doing so, the sign of the cross is imprinted into circulation when man takes hold of the body with spirit and soul in the first breath.

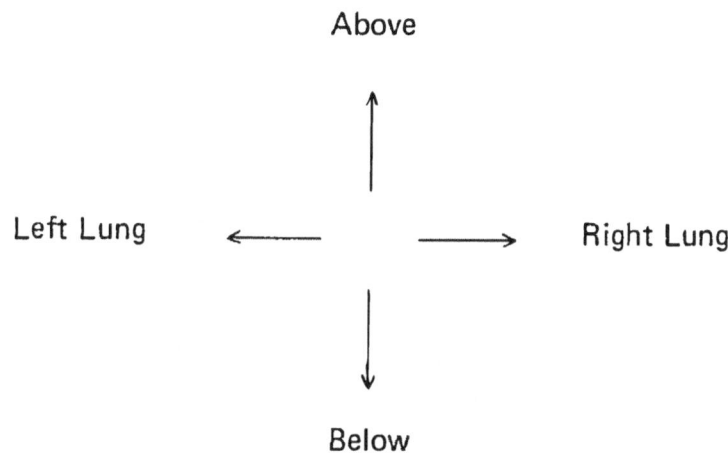

In the lectures *Ways to a New Style in Architecture*,* Rudolf Steiner describes the heavenly archetype of circulation as the relationship between the great heavenly bodies Sun, Moon, and Earth. Man as microcosm has in his world of organs his inner world system. The forces which for the macrocosm proceed from the planets, proceed for the microcosm man from the center of the inner organs. All ancient cultures possessed this knowledge. It was still known by the sages of the Middle Ages, the last of whom was probably Paracelsus, who out of the vestiges of clairvoyant knowledge provided the organs with celestial names.

Thus the heart is our inner Sun, the brain our inner Moon, the lungs our inner Earth. By developing lungs, spirit and soul can advance to a fully human incarnation and act upon earth. The relationships of the lungs to the element earth, to climate and soil consistency are well known. They may be exposed to cold without becoming ill, like no other organ. And finally let us realize that from the lungs there proceed forces which in nutrition bring about the formation of human physical bodily substance. The failure of these forces leads to the illness we call 'consumption.' The lung is then no longer able to build up earthly substance.

---

*   Rudolf Steiner Press, London, 1927.

The Moon is the cosmic mirror without its own life, reflecting the universe. Our inner moon, the brain, is the mirror for our consciousness, comprising all impressions and likewise able to mirror the whole world for this consciousness.

Circulation thus repeats the great world in its effective interrelationships and copies it in the microcosm. Its center is the inner sun, and the *rhythm* that pulsates through breathing and circulation is a *cosmic sun rhythm*.

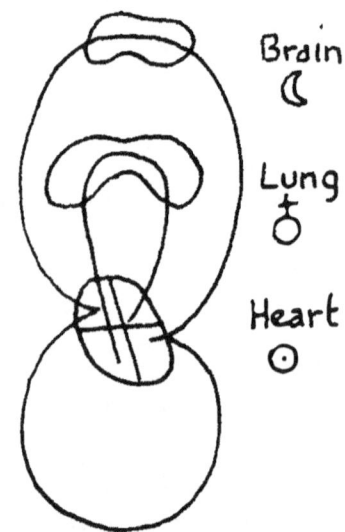

Archetype of Circulation

We count on the average eighteen breaths and seventy-two pulse beats a minute. In twenty-four hours we breathe 25,920 times. It takes the same number of years for the vernal point of the sun—the point on the ecliptic at which the sun rises on March 21st—to journey once through the zodiac. This period is called the Platonic cosmic year. Thus we are tied in our rhythmical system to the mysteries of the sun's passage through the zodiac. Here where we open ourselves in the lung directly to the surrounding world it instills a rhythm into us which shows us to be a being whose life is connected with the sun force of the universe. This rhythm of breath and pulse finds itself placed, as already stated, into the polarity of the upper and lower processes whereby the upper are the formative, but also the hardening and breaking-down processes of the sense-nerve system, the lower the warming and loosening building-up processes of metabolism.

From both sides there may proceed disturbances of the healthy heart function. Rudolf Steiner has given a most descriptive and simple common denominator for the individually very complicated conditions of the heart. This facilitates the comprehension of the pathological states of the heart. He explained how the heart either resists circulation, is obstinate, as it were, or surrenders too much to circulatory motion. It is obvious at once how, on the one hand, the hardening forces take hold of the heart from above and produce all the variations of angina spasms and their consequences; and on the other hand, the loosening forces produce an excessive slackening and enlargement of the heart muscle. The first instance is the concern of the arterial system, the second instance that of the venous system.

Both tendencies respond well to appropriate treatment through massage.

The arterial system pulsates because in inhalation and the reception of oxygen the astral body takes hold more deeply of the living bloodstream, dips down more deeply and affects the tonus from inside. The arterial pulse wave radiates directly from the systole. The arteries are located deeper in the body than the veins, have a harder wall and incline, therefore, more easily to sclerosis. The left human being is more strongly arterial, the right human being more strongly venous, since here the upper and the lower *vena cava* bring the entire venous blood of the upper man, and from below, through the portal vein and liver, that of the metabolism, to the heart.

The venous blood flows continuously, it is attracted through the life activity of the ether body and is lifted out of gravity into levity. This system is inclined to flaccidity, to withdrawal from the living connection. This produces congestion even to the degree of edema, which is to be considered as the severing of fluids from the life connections, and furthermore secondary inflammations and similar phenomena.

Since the living hand can itself activate the formative systole and the sucking diastole through varying the quality of the grip the field of circulatory disturbances, which is the beginning of many illnesses, is one of those fields where Rhythmic Massage can be a direct help to the deteriorating functions. At the periphery the hand can carry out a kind of second heart activity. The peripheral heart activity starts where the pulse wave dies away in the capillary field. This rhythmical warming and enlivening of the periphery is able effectively to relieve the heart activity in every respect. The questions to be considered and the dangers to be avoided will be dealt with in another part of this book.

9.

METAMORPHOSES OF THE SKELETON

In order to recognize the human body as an image of the macrocosm, as a form that can be given to man only by the highest member of his being, by the ego, it is necessary to observe the skeleton in the Goetheanistic sense.

Lavater writes in his *Physiognomic Fragments*: 'It may have been noted that I consider the bony system as the basic design of man, the skull as the fundamental of the bony system, and all flesh merely the coloring of this design.'

Goethe, too, acknowledges the bony structure to be the distinct framework of all forms, which if clearly recognized facilitates the recognition of all the remaining parts. Indeed, he treats the bones as a text to which everything living and human may be joined. Thus we too may feel the importance these researchers attribute to the comprehension of the riddle of the skeleton.

A ground plan must show the character of the architect. What confronts us as human body is not a form that could ever be given to us by the physical forces of the earth. It is the body temple built for man according to the laws of the spirit, of the ego of man. If the spirit leaves its vessel, the latter falls rapidly to dust.

Rudolf Steiner once formulated the sentence: 'The physical body is the hieroglyph of the cosmos.' It is, thus, an image of the contracted being of the whole cosmos. The divine spirit created man in its image. This is the mighty text that Goethe tried to decipher from the language of the skeleton. What Goethe began, Rudolf Steiner unfolds to full survey, making the text readable for us. The scope of this book allows only a short glance at the general relationships in order to understand the structure of the physical body in connection with the members of man's being.

The skeleton stands before us, four-membered. Skull, chest, and limbs are collectively held together and placed into earthly space by the spinal column. The same connection results if we say: spirit, soul, and life, or, related to man in the language of Spiritual Science: ego, astral body, and ether body (life body) are carried into earthly space through being bound to the physical body. The physical body, the fundamental design of which is the skeleton, shows the same membering. The skull in particular is shaped by the ego, the chest space by the soul, the metabolic-limb part by the life processes. All three are placed into space by the metamorphosing principle of the vertebrae.

The vertebra, pictorially spoken the salt cube, was from the very beginning, if we proceed from the physical plane, considered the key to the whole. Oken already said: "The whole bony system is nothing but a repeated vertebra." And Lavater states that he experiences, ever and again, new pleasure and joy in becoming aware of the ever more astonishing, more beautiful and more surprising carrying out of that simple theme of the vertebra.

The vertebra thus is the bone of bones, the archetype to use Goethe's expression, but already the archetype in the contracted Sal-state, through the forces of the physical plane. The actual archetype is always a supersensible, imaginative picture, as was Goethe's archetypal plant which Schiller called 'only an idea.' Goethe's slightly annoyed answer to this was that he was glad to be able to see his ideas with his eyes.

The true archetype of the whole skeleton, clearly defined by the ego, becomes visible if one bases it upon the lemniscate, the form ascribed to the sun in the cosmos, harmonizing all polarities. To make the matter more easily understood, I shall use some diagrams from the articles by Karl König, who occupied himself with this theme, published in the magazine *Natura*, now out of print (IV, Nos. 6 & 7, V, Nos. 1 & 12).

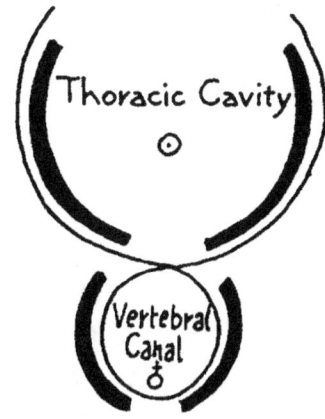

Lemniscate of the Archetype of Vertebra and Rib

Man is a creation of the middle, between cosmos and earth. Also the lemniscate is developed most distinctly and clearly in the middle region of the skeleton, in the middle of the thorax. Karl König here quotes Rudolf Steiner, who describes in a lecture that the form of loops ordinarily called the apparent forms of movement of the planets, is a basic structural form of the human organism. Its perfect expression is to be found in the vertebra-rib system. Vertebra and rib belong together; born out of the cosmos, representing the archetype of the skeletal metamorphoses. Functionally, the lemniscate forms in its upper loop a so-called *sun space* and in its lower loop an *earth space*.*

---

* See George Adams: *The Plant between Sun and Earth*, Goethean Science Foundation, Clent, 1952.) Here the chest space enclosed by the ribs and opening toward the cosmos represents the sun space, the vertebra the contracted earth space. The sun space open to the cosmic forces contains the sun organ heart, the contracted earth space the spinal cord, a moon organ.

This knowledge sheds a confirming light upon the wisdom-filled imaginative language of the Bible. It was not possible to create Eve out of the earthly contracted vertebra, but she was created out of the rib that had remained in a plastic etheric state.

In addition it becomes clear, since the two spaces correspond to a lemniscate, that also rib and vertebra must correspond to one another. The motif of the formation of the rib must return transformed in the vertebra.

The trinitarian motif of the formation of the human shape is a threefold systole and diastole, contraction and expansion. Goethe considered node and leaf the simplest motif for the plant, which only unites an ether body with its physical body. The motif must be sounded three times in man, who has to unite soul and spirit to the formations of the physical body.

The rib, therefore, is still a hovering formation, flowing along musically like a melody and revealing the etheric more than the form of the vertebra adapted to space.

Rib and vertebra are built as follows:

Rib	**Vertebra**
1. Head	1. Corpus
2. Neck	2. Arcus
3. Tubercle	3. Processus transversus
4. Intermediate piece	4. Processus articularis superior
5. Angle	5. Processus articularis inferior
6. Shaft	6. Processus spinalis

These are three contractions and three expansions. They find themselves again in contracted form in the vertebra, which thereby signifies a first metamorphosis of this etheric rib melody downward into the physical and spatial realm.

In principle we may say that metamorphoses of an archetype arise when this archetype is taken hold of by different worlds of forces. Up to now we have seen the archetype in its etheric and physical formation. The question now arises as to the result if soul and spirit, astral body and ego, take hold of the lemniscatic archetype, that is to say, of the vertebra-rib system.

Perhaps it may be stated beforehand that within this system of vertebra and rib there are no metamorphoses upward and downward, but only variations that are determined in the upward direction by etheric forces, in the downward direction by physical forces of gravity. The uppermost vertebra is but a rib-ring (Atlas), the lowest but a vertebra cube.

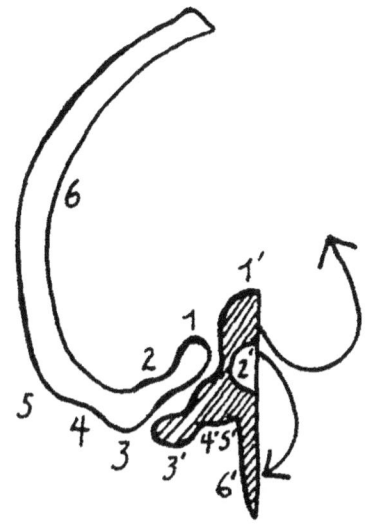

Transformation of Rib into Vertebra

In dealing with the skeleton we quite involuntarily use musical concepts that characterize the facts most distinctly. This lies in the nature of music, for music is the harmony of the spheres made earthly. It contains the cosmic orders of the universe which in the microcosm man are represented by his ego. The musical laws are of the rank of the ego. We shall come back to this in our discussion of the spinal column.

In dealing with the question of how soul and spirit take hold of the archetype of the skeleton, I shall draw upon a further presentation of Goethe's where he demonstrates upon another artistic field a living cosmic order. This is his *Theory of Color*. It is not in vain that Goethe considered his *Theory of Color* the most significant of his productions, higher even than his dramas. Seen from the point of view of the modern Science of the Spirit, it reveals, in contrast to Newton's theory of color, the ascent from a mechanical to a cosmically living order mirroring the formative laws of the etheric world. From an indifferent listing of colors Goethe awakens them to a relationship with soul and spirit.

I should like to place two diagrams side by side. (See diagram next page)

Goethe takes the starting point from the two pure colors, yellow and blue, representing light and darkness, and as colors containing nothing from each other. *These pure polarities mix themselves downward into green*. Green is a denser color, supportive and harmonious, that likes to limit itself. It is the color of the living earth. We step gladly upon green, in blue we would drown, red would constantly excite us. For soul experience Goethe follows the same procedure we followed in considering the skeleton when two ribs, an absolute polarity in their form, by condensation metamorphose themselves into a vertebra. Goethe calls the triangle which thus forms itself the triangle of nature, and the physical-etheric shape of the vertebra-rib is related to the vegetative forms.

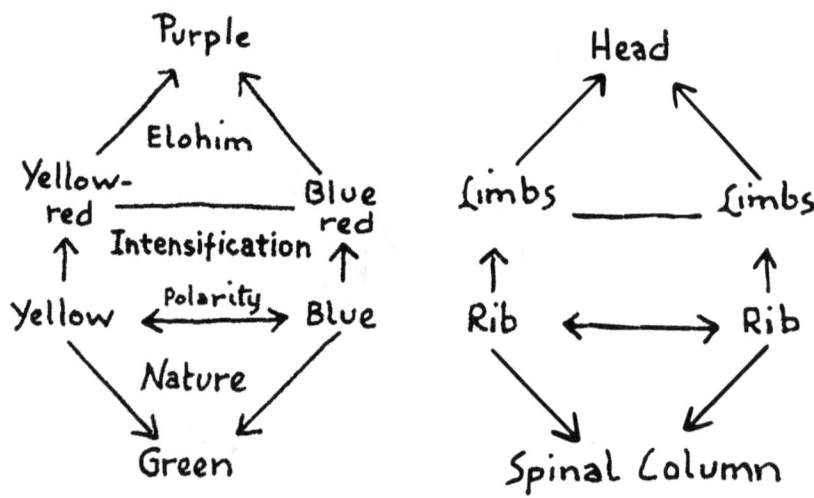

Now Goethe introduces the concept of *intensification*, of inner exertion. An urging soul element expresses itself therein, the beginning of an *evolution*. Thereby he comes to red as a new color quality. Red is activity, the dramatic element in the world of colors, bearing evolution as does the soul-astral element.

In the color spectrum there appears on the one side yellow-red with its radiating character, on the other side blue-red with the character of shining inward, of inwardness.

If the astral body of man takes hold of the archetype, the limbs come into existence. The rib in its development can be experienced musically, as Rudolf Steiner indicates in eurythmy, the art of movement. Proceeding from the keynote, as it were, the limb develops in a formation similar to the musical scale: upper arm, lower arm, wrist, fingers, and so forth. Not only the etheric element but the starry cosmos takes hold of the shaping of the rib out of the planetary world of forces, out of the astra.—I am drawing here only a sketch, more detailed elaborations are possible; they would, however, go beyond the scope of this book.—Through such a consideration a strong light can be shed upon the shape and inner significance of the limbs as expression of our soul and capacity of motion. We turn outward in the major mood, inward in the minor mood. This comes to expression in the skeleton through supination and pronation. *A limb is an unfurled rib.* Its middle, knee and elbow, are sun places in polar differentiation upward and downward, just as in the cosmos what is above and what is below the sun confront each other. The relationships of knee and elbow to the sun or the ego, indeed to the heart, are easily to be understood.

Finally, with Goethe, the whole is crowned in purple as *higher synthesis*, not downward as in green in a condensation of substance, but *upward* in immaterial permeation of yellow-red and blue-red. This crowning of purple corresponds to the head in man's formation. When the ego brings about the final and highest comprehension of the whole skeleton the head can come into existence, appearing in cosmic-spherical form, purple in the character of its formation, simultaneously beginning and end, crown and seed. For the cosmos does not, as we do, build with single stones, but it begins with the whole. In the embryo the head is formed first, the other parts follow.

Since in the formation of the skeleton, according to the biogenetic fundamental law, all stages of man's development must be repeated, the real process is of great and sublime complication. We shall comprehend it completely only if we study the evolution of macrocosm and microcosm from a point of view different from the usual one, that is to say, from the point of view of astronomy and embryology, side by side. In justifiable anticipation of the creative force behind the nuances of red in the world of color, Goethe called the upper triangle formed by yellow-red, blue-red, and purple, the *triangle of the Elohim*, the form-creating divinity, in the Science of the Spirit called 'Spirits of Form.' They are, in truth, the creators of the world and the protectors of the human ego.

We have tried here through artistic feeling to find our way to the essential nature of these processes that are never grasped without reverence. Goethe's great achievement in his *Theory of Color* can be comprehended when we in this way discover that he really demonstrates the formative laws of the etheric world for the interaction of light and darkness. From this viewpoint we comprehend that the physical body is the vessel for the ego-spirit or light-spirit descending into darkness.

$$
\begin{array}{cc}
\text{Head} & \text{Ego} \\
\uparrow & \\
\text{Limbs} & \text{Astral Body} \\
\uparrow & \\
\text{Ribs} & \text{Ether Body} \\
\uparrow & \\
\text{Spinal Column} & \text{Physical Body}
\end{array}
$$

Metamorphosis of the Basic Form
through the Members of Man's Being

10.

THE MUSCLE SYSTEM

Muscle system, bone system, and nerve system find their inception as early as the third week of pregnancy, when beside the chorda dorsalis the 44 pairs of primal vertebral-cell conglomerations come into being. This is the time when ego and astral body join with the germ and induce, working out of the sheaths, this first inception of their tools. Simultaneously, even somewhat earlier, blood circulation and the inception of the heart become visible.

Considered from the spiritual-scientific viewpoint, *nerve system* and *muscle system* are a *creation of the astral body* that provides beings with consciousness and motion.

The nerve system is the star-like constructed image of the astral body. When it is completed in space, the astral body withdraws from it and uses it from outside as its instrument for the formation of consciousness, as is described in the chapter on blood and nerves.

On the other hand, the muscle system, strongly permeated by blood, appears as though congealed out of the living fluid organism. We are reminded of this by the fish-like muscles about which we speak instinctively of head (*caput*), abdomen, and tail (*cauda*). Here the astral body is submerged throughout life and permeates the entire muscle system with impulses of motion. The muscle system is, as it were, hung up on the skeleton. The protein substance, capable of contraction, makes it possible that the astral body carries out in it a kind of *submerged breathing* movement, by connecting itself more deeply in the contraction and again loosening itself in the relaxation, causing a transformation of substance that expresses itself in an acid formation, as is the case in every stronger interference of the astral body. In breathing it is carbonic acid, in muscles it is lactic acid. Today one knows the course of the waves of contraction through the muscle fibres in the most minute details. Three hundred or more times per second such a wave courses through the fibres of the skeletal muscles. One sees how the astral body glimmers, as it were, through the muscles and produces the tonus, the muscle tone. The middle state between the extremes of cramp and flaccidity is the healthy one. The rhythm between taking hold of the muscles and letting go must be possible in order to have a normal course of motion.

The muscular system, too, is part of the threefold being. First we have *striated muscles* which enfold, as it were, the bony system, mostly in three layers which at the extremities are normally sheared against each other. In the trunk the outer layers are large; nearer the bones, the muscles, especially in the back, become small, minute formations.

The so-called striation rests upon a different light refraction of the protein; it is thus a light structure as a result of the astral body's weaving through the muscle. The dark part of the fibre is the contractile part. When the astral body takes hold of the muscle the protein passes over from a more fluid, so-called *Sol state* into a denser, gelatinous *Gel state* which must at once be dissolved again with the relaxation of the muscle into the more fluid Sol state. We can move muscles of this structure arbitrarily.

Secondly, we have the *smooth muscles* belonging to the metabolic region. They enfold the hollow organs such as intestine, stomach, bladder, uterus, and so on, but are also to be found in other places such as blood vessels, skin, glandular organs wherever movement of some kind is needed. These are the movements we are not aware of and which we do not control. These muscles consist of spindle shaped cells, they have more nuclei, are more capable of regeneration and more lively. Their movements are slower, have a worm-like contraction, and are, on the other hand, more continuous. The smooth muscle fibres do not have the light character of the striation but they are marked by the watery-etheric element. The bundled form of the fibres is relieved through interwoven textures as they are found in lower plants.

The *heart muscle* is the third element lying between the two and forming a special type. It unites elements of both sides and is partially striated. Nevertheless, with the exception of very few human beings, we are unable to influence the heart activity arbitrarily. In their case it is the result of training. The striation, however, indicates that in the future men can and will become more conscious of the heart function. In the heart there exists a bridge, present nowhere else, between nerve and muscle inasmuch as the autonomous nerve system of the heart, the so-called conducting system, continues in the muscles and presents an intermediary between nerve fibre and muscle fibre in its anatomical structure.

The drawing on the page opposite, already known, may further elucidate the relationship of the muscle system to the members of man's being. The lemniscate again represents the astral body and the ego. The systems of nerves and bones are formed by the upper astral body and ego and then by stages released into mineralization. Polarically opposed to this is the system of muscles and the blood which are shaped by the submerged part of astral body and ego. In bones and blood the most dead confronts the most living.—It goes without saying that this is a mere scheme for the general situation. In the lower man the two higher members are 'incarnated.'

The muscle system is constantly permeated and woven through by the astral body that is taken into the body by the first breath. As already mentioned the astral body produces the tone, the tension, the constant unrest that at once appears if the upper pole does not control the motive power of the lower one. Here, too, man is a being of balance. I repeat: the muscular motion, the single systole and diastole of every fibre may be viewed as a submerged breathing. What the astral body does in breathing, the soft dipping into the blood, the forming of carbonic acid and the exhalation as a releasing process, it does in intensified manner in motion deeper down in the organic processes. It dips down more strongly into the muscle, also forms an acid as a result of its activity; namely, lactic acid, and then emerges again, is released or, expressed more clearly, is driven out by the etheric body. Recall the saying of the alchemists: the element water 'drives out, expels.' (See the chapter, 'The Warmth Organism'). This breathing process of motion has, to be sure, fallen away from the cosmic sun order of the rhythmic system into the sphere of willing which, insofar as we use it, is subject to our arbitrary will and on the other hand is dependent upon metabolism. It is, however, chiefly a rhythmical process that has two pathological final states: cramp and complete flaccidity.

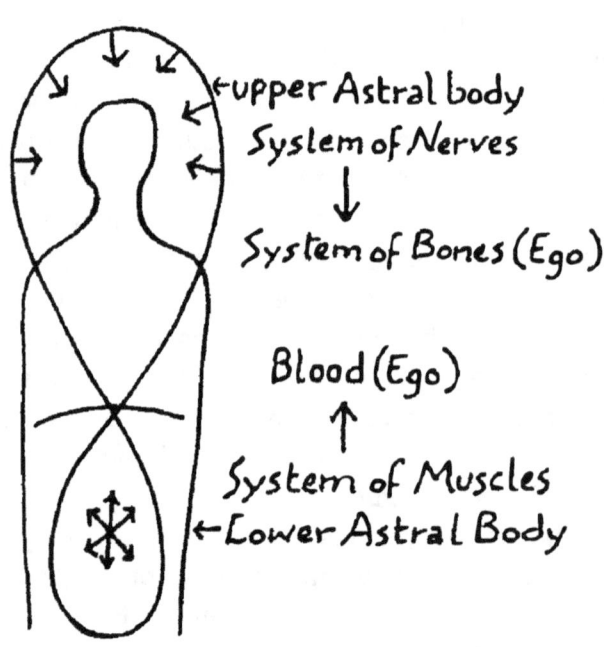

We can observe in the little child how the metabolic processes pass over into processes of motion. Indeed, we can conclude from its happily kicking movements that a baby has a healthy metabolism. These first, seemingly chaotic, movements are only gradually directed by consciousness and made sure of their aim by the ego. Here the upper man already gives the directive.

The lower astral body would constantly carry out its impulses of motion in the muscles if the upper astral body were not to intervene from above via the nervous system, calming and restraining. If it does not do so there arise through a morbid nervous system unconscious processes of motion such as tics, trembling and seizures of the limbs up to the most serious agitations such as St. Vitus' dance.

The other extreme is paralysis. To make this clear I should like to quote a passage from the book by Rudolf Steiner and Ita Wegman: *Fundamentals of Therapy*:*

> "Observe the transition from the painful movement of a limb to its paralysis. In the movement accompanied by pain we have the initial stages of a movement paralyzed. . . . We actuate a certain idea, and the movement of a limb ensues. We do not enter consciously with the idea into the organic processes which culminate in the movement. The idea dives down into the unconscious. Between the idea and the movement an act of feeling intervenes; but this—in the healthy condition—works in the soul only, it does not attach itself distinctly to any bodily organic processes. In disease, however, it is different. The feeling, experienced in health as a thing distinct and apart, unites with the physical organization in the conscious experience of illness . . .
>
> . . . There must be something there which, when the body is in health, is less intensely united with it than when it is diseased. To spiritual perception this 'something' is revealed to be the astral body. The astral body is a supersensible organization within that which the senses can perceive. If it takes hold of an organ only loosely, it leads to an inner experience of soul, an experience which subsists in itself and is not felt to be in connection with the body. If, on the other hand, the astral body takes hold of an organ strongly or intensely, it leads to the consciousness of illness . . .
>
> . . . Spiritual perception finds beside the astral body a special ego organization which lives and expresses itself with freedom of soul in thought. If with the ego organization man takes intense hold of his bodily nature, the ensuing condition makes his observation of his own organism similar to that of the external world.
>
> . . . In a human limb this condition only takes place when it is paralyzed. The limb then becomes a piece of outer world. The ego organization is no longer loosely united with it as it is in health, when it can unite with the limb in the act of movement and withdraw again at once. It dives down into the limb permanently and is no longer able to withdraw."

The healthy movement, the movement accompanied by pain, and paralysis, are stages of the penetration of the astral body and the ego into the organic processes. If

---

*   Rudolf Steiner Press, London, 1967.

no loosening can take place paralysis is complete. Spasms and cramps are concomitant disturbances on this course of action with a predominant astral body.

The way movement arises organically is quite a different question which we shall also try to make clear.

Every movement with conscious aim needs for its realization the interplay of the entire functions of threefold man.

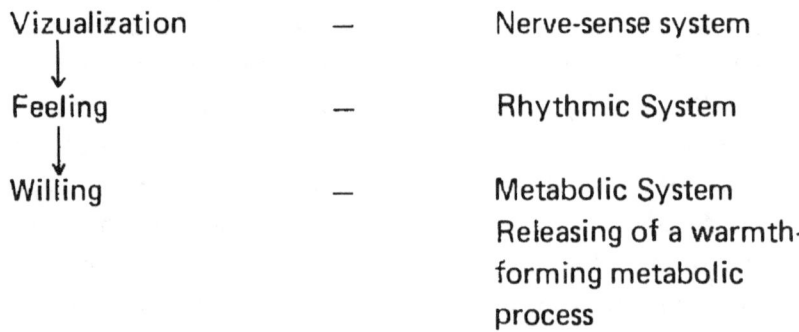

Every muscle attached to the bone has its nerve and an excellent blood supply. The motor-nerve system mediates the perception of the muscle to the ego.

The thought (visualization) passes into the unconscious via a feeling, that is, a rhythmical process.

The metabolic process gives to the ego the possibility, through the *formation of warmth*, of taking hold of the muscular system, of *actually carrying out* the movement.

If I cut the nerve, I am no longer inwardly connected with the muscle, it is outer world for my consciousness, like a book that lies on the table, and I cannot move. If I make the muscle bloodless, I cannot move it either, because the warmth process is lacking by means of which the ego has really to take hold of it. The carried out movement I perceive in all its phases.

The nervous system has perceptive character only. With the realization of the will the spirit takes immediate hold of the organism on the basis of a warmth process, not, however, the visualizing part of the spirit but the part of the spirit that has incarnated bodily. Our body is pervaded by spirit and soul. Psychologists call this entire field 'the unconscious.' The unconscious, however, is of a spirit-soul nature. The lower loop in our drawing points to the fact that there exists a part of our soul and of our spirit that works bodily. This part is connected with our inner cosmos, with the inverted world of organs; it contains deep secrets which we are only beginning to investigate. This aspect of the problem of motion leads us to questions of destiny, to the question of freedom of will or bondage.—The following may be said: The actual mover is the spirit, we move in our space of destiny. This destiny rests concealed in us, at times premonitions arise. It leads us to encounters, to happy and painful experiences whose meaning lies in our destiny. At incarnation, the soul carries the spirit deeply into the body and it serves the spirit also in the system of motions, for our gestures, for example, are a language that is able to reveal much of the character of our spirit and soul.

In every movement all the four members of our being participate. *The ego provides the certainty of goal*, the directive power. *The astral body places the movement correctly into space.* The plant, not possessing an astral body, is indifferent as to the position in space of its parts, it is attracted from outside by the light. Cosmic forces bestow upon it aim and direction from outside. Man himself gives aim and direction to his movements; he carries his body through life properly inserted into the spatial forces.

The ether of life body gives shape to movement, beautiful or angular, artistic or stiff. It is the sculptor that shapes the character of the higher members of our being in movement.

And through the physical body man develops the force of carrying out the movement. Everything works together and joins into a whole.

When Goethe in viewing Greek sculpture speaks of 'grace and dignity,' he expresses thereby that the Greeks presented the shapes of their Gods and heroes in no other way but with gestures showing how spirit and soul form and control the body in heavenly order and balance. No overpowering form outside, no passion from inside distorts the gesture that can be beautiful because the Divine shines through it. They rest in themselves, 'void of destiny,' as it was felt by Hölderlin.

From the breathing interplay of the members of man's being in the system of muscles it becomes evident that this system, coagulated, as it were, from the man of fluids, in connection with skin and subcutaneous tissue, is the main field of treatment through Rhythmical Massage.

Any treatment through massage takes hold of the equilibrium between upper and lower man through binding and releasing of spirit and soul in relationship to the body. This was Hippocrates' conception of gymnastics and massage, that is to say, active and passive movement as described in the chapter, 'The History of Massage' concerning the differentiated binding and loosening.

Since the diving down and emerging of the members of man's being takes place through a rhythmical process of which we are only slightly conscious, Rhythmical Massage is beneficial and harmonizing for all anomalies of motion through the very fact that it renders the breathing interplay underlying every movement more fluid, stimulates the metabolism of the muscle, permeates it with gentle or strong consciousness, both poles harmoniously uniting in rhythm.

Flaccidity and paralysis, nutritional disturbance and atrophy, spasms and hardening are treated through changes in the quality of the grip and direction of motion. It becomes immediately evident that any application of mechanical forces must disturb the living interplay.

The masseur must make his own the thought that, if soul and spirit normally move the muscles from inside, his grip from outside must possess the same living, ensouled and mindful character, so that his massage may call forth an echo in the inner life. One might say: The way I address the tissues, the same way they answer. One calls forth the individual activity of the patient, allures, as it were, the soul and spirit of the patient gradually to take over the disturbed function himself. This is a general principle of Rhythmical Massage which we shall deal with in another chapter.

11.

THE INNER WORLD SYSTEM

The cosmic, astral forces that act in the plant from outside and differentiate and shape its life processes have become inner forces in man, who is the bearer of a soul. He has, therefore, an organism that must build up an organic inner world. So the world of organs must be called an *inner world system*. Whereas sun, moon and planets act upon the plant from outside, the corresponding astral forces in the microcosm have their centers in the inner organs and, radiating from there, control the life processes of the human body. The organs thus correspond to an *inverted planetary system*. All the form impulses for the physical body spring from the zodiac. The last, decadent remains of a once wisdom-filled comprehension of these relationships we have in the fact that we allot certain regions of the physical body to the various signs of the zodiac: the head to the Ram, the neck region to Taurus, the arms to the Twins, and so forth. Today, however, this is a completely external tradition no longer understood. For we are here concerned with twelve mighty form impulses or form gestures that have been described by Rudolf Steiner.* To describe them here in detail would lead us too far. The organic life that fills the body is allotted to the planetary system. We have thus an inner world system. In describing blood circulation we have already pointed to this fact. In order to elucidate the connection of the organs and their treatment we shall once more deal with this inner world system.

Circulation, with the heart as the co-ordinating sun organ, is the basis for the inner world system just as it is the sun in the macrocosm that collects the system around itself. We might even say that the sun forces are modified through the planetary forces, above the sun and below the sun, and what once was an all-embracing unity has through a long evolutionary process differentiated itself and unfolded sevenfold.

In the plant, receiving the effects of the stars from outside, we find the influence of the moon activity in the development of the root, we then rise through Mercury and Venus to the formation of leaf and blossom. The effects of the planets above the sun, Saturn, Jupiter and Mars, are to be found in the formation of fruit and seed. Since the vegetative functional aspect of the plant is inverted in man through the insertion of soul and spirit, we find it in man in reverse order.

The inner *moon* organ corresponding in the plant to the realm of the root we find in man above in the head. It is the *brain* with its mirroring force mediating consciousness.

---

* See lecture given by Rudolf Steiner in Dornach on October 28, 1921, published in 1972 by Rudolf Steiner Verlag, Dornach, as Lecture Fifteen in *Anthroposophie als Kosmosophie*, Part II.

From this sphere the tendencies of mineralization and materialization radiate into the rest of the organism. Further down, we find the inner *Mercury*, the *lungs*, whose activity corresponds to the breathing leaf region in the plant. There follows in man the *kidney* as inner *Venus*, the region that corresponds in the plant to the blossom, connected with the whole system of reproduction that is deeply embedded in the blood process. The blood 'blossoms' in this way, it evaporates, it contains the tendency of continually passing over from the physical into the etheric. It must be constantly renewed. The kidney, with its structure resembling the calyx of a plant and with its thousands of little glomeruli blossoms of red blood, suggests to an imaginative, artistic observation the relationship to the blossom region of the plant. Rudolf Steiner speaks of 'kidney radiation' which is another expression for the activity of the astral body in the kidney that permeates the whole metabolism with astrality and is light-related like a kind of higher, metamorphosed blossom-radiation. Indeed, the kidney, our inner Venus, is described by Rudolf Steiner as an inner light-producing organ.

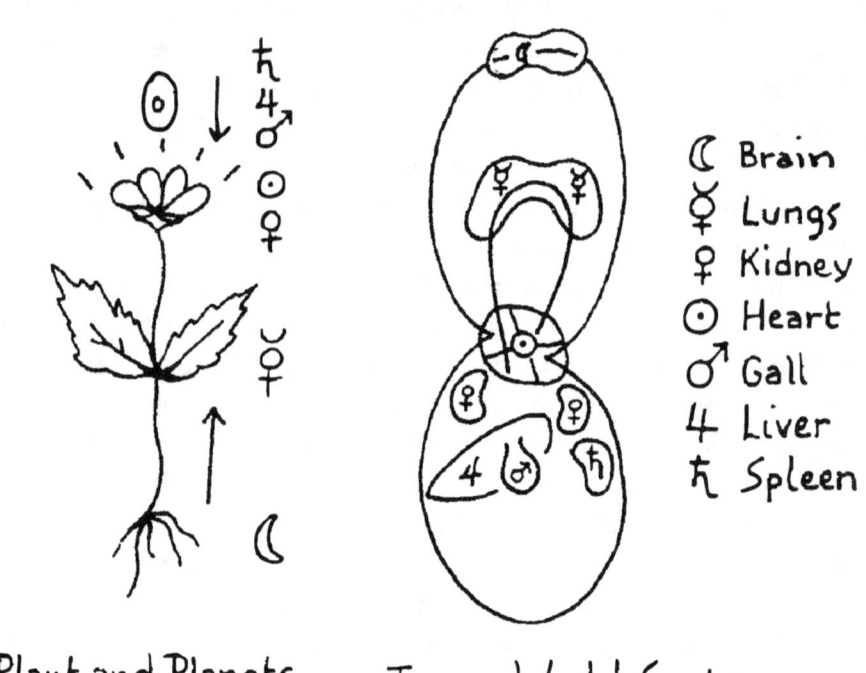

Plant and Planets   Inner World System

The three great organs, *spleen*, *liver*, and *gall*, belong to the lower circulation; they have to do with the building up and with the inner metabolic processes that correspond to the fruit and seed formation in the plant. They are our inner Saturn, Jupiter, and Mars. The spleen, the inner Saturn organ, has in regard to the microcosm man a task similar to that of the outermost planet Saturn, who like a guardian circles around the solar system and has to change and harmonize with the rhythms of the solar system all the effects from outside of the zodiac and the rest of the universe. The spleen fulfills for the microcosm man the same task in metabolism. It must equalize all irregularities and foreign rhythms in the substances of nutrition. This activity is carried out by the ether body of the spleen. The spleen itself may even be removed without detrimental effect upon man.

We must call the liver, our inner Jupiter, the wisdom-filled alchemist. It controls the entire field of substances. Here organic substances are built up, broken down, reconstructed, freed of poison, mobilized, and stored. These are processes that bear witness to the unending wisdom of the astral and ego organization belonging to the liver. The gall, the inner Mars, does not contain physical iron, but it contains the Mars secret of binding the spiritual to the physical. This inner Mars sees to it that the forces of the ego, of the individuality, penetrate right into the physical, and that the entire metabolism remains accessible not only to the astral but also to the activity of the ego.

All these activities are only one aspect of the much more comprehensive tasks that the organs accomplish for the whole organism.

Paracelsus was the last to apply the planetary names to the organs. Rudolf Steiner was the first to verify them again, not from ancient traditions but from his modern spiritual research. We still have to explain why the kidney as subsolar organ does not lie above the diaphragm like the other two subsolar organs. Here we have to turn to important evolutionary facts. The kidney's inception takes place by stages far above in the embryo (archetypal kidney, pre-kidney, and so forth). It is a descending organ. Its gradual transformation accompanies the descent of the entelechy man from an existence in the supersensible in full harmony with the solar cosmos (described in the Bible as Paradise and portrayed in the picture of the Expulsion from Paradise) into an existence in physical bodies on the earth for the development, through resistance, of the ego, of the free individuality. Previously, man was a light-breather, now he becomes an air-breather. According to the ontogenetic law of Haeckel, the embryo must show traces of this development. The kidney, so closely connected with breathing and ensouling, descends and becomes united with the region of metabolism. The astral body can no longer only play around the blossom as in the case of the plant, it must through the development of air breathing dive into the body and work, radiating from the kidney, into the entire region of metabolism. Seen imaginatively and artistically, the kidney is a materialized blossom, caught in the arterial blood stream that absorbs the full incarnating impact of inhalation and leads it further in the organization. This submerged part of the astral body manifests in the transformation of red blood into blue blood, in the forming of carbonic acid. On the other hand the liver, our inner cosmic laboratory of transformation of substances, is inserted into the blue bloodstream of the portal vein. When it has completed its work, circulation leads the blood to the right heart where exhalation is prepared and at the same time the disengaging, the partial excarnation.

Again we meet Goethe's two blessings:

> 'In breathing there are two blessings;
> Draw in the air, release it again,
> The first compresses, the second refreshes;
> Thus marvellous is the mixture of life.
> Give thanks to God when he presses you
> And thank him when he releases you.'

The functioning of the human organism, entangled and many-layered, can only be sketchily described, in order to build up a more living image of the total functioning. We see the soul and spirit in man build up a body in the image of 'God,' in the image of the 'universe' if the latter is considered the body of the Divine.

The functions of the individual organs and the indications for treatment with Rhythmical Massage will be dealt with for every single organ concerned in the chapter, 'Massage for the Organs.'

12.

THE SKIN

The observation of the skin as an important organ of life belongs to the most informative experiences of the masseur.

As a totality the skin belongs to the nerve-sense system since it develops, like the latter, from the outer germinal layer and is the bearer of extensive sensory experience. With its various layers it is at the same time representing the organism as a whole. In this connection the skin is in a special position. Since it enfolds the entire organism, limiting thereby all inner processes of this microcosm, we have to recognize in it a field in which the formative forces of the all-embracing *ego* are especially active. Man's figure is a *spirit-figure*, it is his *ego-figure*. The ego as the highest of all forces must draw all the differentiations together into a sum total and must finally bring about harmony. In the skin of the white race this shows even in the appearance of the peach blossom color. The complexion is the result of the transformation of light. The peach blossom, Goethe's dissolved purple, is the highest harmony between the active and passive side of colors, between light and darkness.

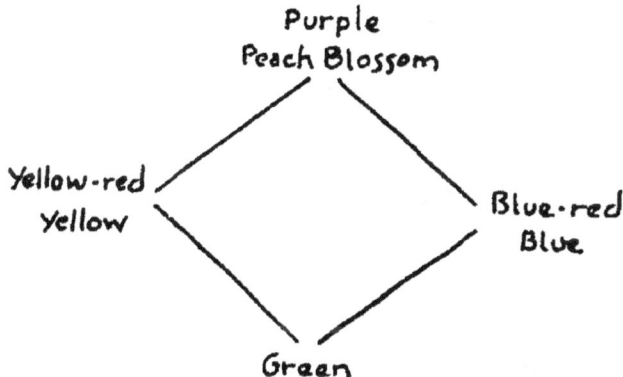

The appearance of different shades of color in the skin, for instance greenish, indicates the withdrawal of the ego as in nausea, and the welling up of vegetative processes. The appearance of blue-reddish color indicates inner congestions.

There are special indications by Rudolf Steiner from which it becomes evident that also the contour of the races is a question of light digestion and absorption.*

As representative of the organism as a whole, the skin shows a threefold structure. Outside it participates in the nerve-sense activity which inside is joined by the metabolism in the subcutaneous tissues. In between we find a zone of the capillary field in which rhythmical processes, such as breathing and circulation, predominate. The following sketch will illustrate these relationships showing the layers of skin which mirror in detail the seven great life processes within the threefold membering.

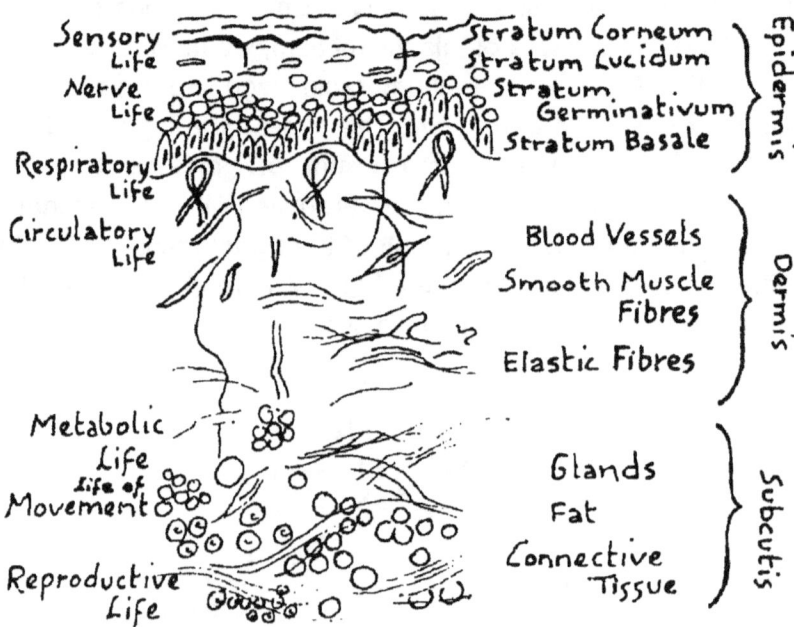

In the skin from outside inwards all the great life functions are represented which Rudolf Steiner described as *seven stages of life*; that is to say, different stages of etheric life activity:**

1. The Life of Senses
2. The Life of Nerves

---

*   Lecture, Dornach, March 3, 1923.
** See lectures given by Rudolf Steiner in Dornach on October 29, 1921 (published in 1972 by Rudolf Steiner Verlag, Dornach, as Lecture Sixteen in *Anthroposophie als Kosmosophie. Zweiter Teil*).

3. The Life of Respiration
4. The Life of Circulation
5. The Life of Metabolism
6. The Life of Movement
7. The Life of Reproduction

The *sensory life* in the skin is most advanced toward the outside, for we feel a touching of the skin almost before it takes place. This sensory part of the skin is the outermost boundary of the microcosm. With its millions of point-like nerve endings it makes us think of the view of the outermost limit of the macrocosm, with its innumerable light points. One calls to mind that the nervous system is of cosmic origin and that it was a light structure of the astral body before it took on a solid form. Thus there are countless examples for the truth of the rule of the great Hermes Trismegistos of the Egyptians, the three-times Wise: 'Below everything is as above,' that is to say: the microcosm is built according to the image of the macrocosm.

The life of the senses is followed by the *life of the nerves* which directs the stimulus toward the inside. It makes us able to preserve an impression. If the life of the nerves were lacking, every impression would be extinguished the moment the stimulus of the sense organ ceases.

Still further inward we meet the *life of respiration*. All our impressions finally unload upon breathing. Everybody can experience in himself how breathing vibrates with our content of consciousness.

Breathing, in turn, dips down into *circulation*. This brings us into the center of the life processes and the life stages. From the circulating blood we enter still deeper into the organism. The next stage is the *metabolic life*, the activity of the formation of organs and the binding and dissolving of the earthly substances. The inner alchemy is the activity of the ether body connected with the organs, the fifth stage of life.

This is followed by a further stage, that of the *life of movement*, the force connection in the ether body that serves the movements of the muscles. Finally, we have general *reproduction*.

Thus we have the successive stages of seven life processes that are clearly reflected in the layers of the skin, resulting in a striking parallel.

The epidermis, gradually dying off toward the outside, with its sensory elements, is the place of the life of senses and nerves. It is interesting that in this part there appears a stratum lucidum, a becoming transparent of substance. In the formation of the eye this process is brought to culmination. The skin is a spread-out model of this process. This marks the skin as an organ of light elaboration. Becoming transparent was, for the alchemists, the final and highest stage of substance. The human eye presents organically a degree of perfection of substance that measures up to Goethe's stanza, justifying it: 'If the eye were not sunlike, we would see no light. If God's power did not live in us, (the sunlike spirit of man, the ego) then things divine would give us no delight.'

Thus the skin as a whole is a spread-out eye, exposed to the cosmic radiations. It is, as it were, the guardian for the inner organism. All cosmic forces that surge up to it must either be rejected or, metamorphosed, led to the inner being.

If we summarize all cosmic radiations with the expression 'light,' the skin is the great organ of light breathing and light digestion. An experiment mentioned by Friedrich Husemann in his book *Das Bild des Menschen als Grundlage der Heilkunst,* illustrates the connection between eye and skin. If we irradiate the hindquarters of a frog with light, there appear in the background of its eye changes similar to those caused by direct exposure to light. The outer light, however, must not penetrate into the inner region without transformation. The light digestion reaches right into the metabolic layers of the skin where the pigment is formed and then pushed forward into the layer of the palisade cells, a pre-stage, comparable to the formation of the retina behind which lies the capillary region.—Finally, according to Husemann, all light is transformed into warmth. Thus on the one hand the effects of the cosmic radiations end in the warmth formation, and, on the other hand, all metabolic processes do so likewise. Everything serves the formation of warmth which is the physical basis of the ego, the I, the entelechy Man.

The living skin breathes, and this activity is vital since the loss of more than a third of its surface causes death. From this one can see that there exists a death through suffocation more subtle than that in ordinary breathing. Within certain limits the skin is a protection against rays. It has qualities of detoxification like the kidney which has a special relationship to the skin. The kidney radiation described in the chapter, 'The Inner World System' ends in the skin. If it becomes too strong it causes irritation of the skin. Inflammatory rashes belong to this field. Besides the excretion of urine, the kidney as total organ has a still higher task in the transformation of the absorbed substances of nutrition into man's own protein. The description of this capacity, however, does not belong within the scope of this book. Rudolf Hauschka gives a detailed description in his book *Nutrition.**

The rhythmical part of the skin layers leads us to the metabolic part, the subcutaneous tissues with their glands embedded in loose connective tissue which in the formation of sweat are able to take over some of the work of the kidneys. Here we find also the muscle fibres which are the foundation of the life of motion, and with this part are connected the forces of reproduction for the entire skin.

---

*   Rudolf Hauschka, *Nutrition*, Chapter V, Rudolf Steiner Press, London, 1979.)

If there is a balance between upper and lower processes, a healthy skin will be witness to it. If the nerve-sense processes predominate, the skin becomes too dry, it shrinks and in some cases itches; callosity, scales and even pustules appear. If the dissolving metabolic processes predominate, the skin shows swelling, inflammatory changes, even wet rashes. The symptoms of both sides may mix in complicated skin diseases.

In any case, *skin rashes* are a *contra-indication* for the masseur.

A later chapter will deal with the reason why in Rhythmical Massage oils, possibly with added medication, are used in the care of the skin.

With the Greeks the significance of the skin as personal boundary was well known. Rudolf Steiner draws attention to the difference between the point of view of the Atheneans and that of the Spartans. In the care of the body the Atheneans in every respect took into consideration the living interplay of cosmic influences upon the skin. They permitted light and shadow, warmth and coldness to change in harmonious fashion. The skin thereby remains more penetrable. Indeed, man becomes more inclined to open himself to the surrounding world, to join it socially, and to become communicative.

The Spartans, on the other hand, hardened the skin through rigorous exposure to any weather and through hard manipulation with a mixture of oil and sand. This makes the skin less transparent. It drives all the forces toward the inside. The whole man becomes taciturn, reserved, and of little grace in social relationships. On the other hand, he develops different inner qualities. It goes without saying that with these descriptions no judgments of worth are intended. They show, however, how we can prepare the body in different ways as an instrument of the soul. Today, for instance, the ideal of browning of the skin in full sunlight has a hardening effect upon the inter-relationship of the members of man's being. For since ancient times it has always been considered good and virtuous to keep the balance between the too much and the too little.

From all this it becomes clear that the observation of the skin belongs to the duties of the masseur. His attention is rewarded with the silent and yet so eloquent presentation of the equilibrium of forces in the organism according to its more delicate aspects.

PART TWO

RHYTHMICAL MASSAGE ACCORDING TO DR. ITA WEGMAN

13.

DEVELOPMENT AND ELABORATION

Within the scope of her activity as a physician and in the context of the development of medicine extended through spiritual-scientific knowledge, Dr. Ita Wegman began in the twenties of this century to give special indications for the elaboration of massage according to new directives. At that time, courses for nurses took place at the *Klinisch-Therapeutisches Institut (Clinical-Therapeutic Institute)* in Arlesheim, Switzerland. Dr. Wegman was the founder and principal of this Clinic, and the courses for nurses were inaugurated by Rudolf Steiner himself, though they did not commence till after his death.

All the doctors' assistants, especially of course the nurses, shared instruction in practical, theoretical, and also artistic subjects. The Clinic's college of doctors were the teachers. One of my tasks was the field of massage. Within the scope of these courses, right up to 1940, in twelve years of collaboration with Dr. Wegman whose assistant I was, the fundamentals of a new method of massage were elaborated. In 1940 I returned to Germany where after the war I began to teach this massage in courses. This has continued and been developed further for more than thirty years. The method was termed *Rhythmical Massage According to Dr. Ita Wegman*, because it became necessary to designate it as regards its nature and origin. Since 1962 there has existed in Germany the *School for Artistic Therapy and Massage* in Boll near Göppingen, at the foot of the Swabian Alb.

The classical Swedish massage in which Dr. Wegman herself was trained formed the starting point. The pure fundamental grips of this massage proved to be most suited to transformation in accordance with the new knowledge. At the beginning of the work, Dr. Wegman was present and gave her instructions in every training course. She demonstrated the special manipulations which she considered important. And since she often used me as a model for her demonstrations I was able not only to perceive her intentions from outside, but also to feel inwardly what was especially important in this method of treatment, which rests upon special grip qualities.

The fundamentals of the knowledge of man, inasfar as they come into consideration for massage, have been dealt with in the first part of this book. They were presented in detail in the courses for nurses, since without them a deeper understanding is not possible.

Thus the *fundamental forms* still valid today came into being. These forms or movements have their own inherent laws for the different regions of the body. They can be used as such, or they may be individually transformed for special treatments. This introduces an artistic element into the method, for this process may only be compared with the musical phenomenon of variations on a theme. The fundamental forms are to be compared with the theme, the consciously directed individual treatment with the variations. The Goethean concept of the primeval phenomenon and its metamorphosis may also assist our understanding. A further characteristic is the *emphasis of the rhythmical element* which will be dealt with in another chapter, and also the application of *grips with the quality of suction* rather than the usual quality of pressure. The suction of fluids serves above all the stimulation of the forces of levity that must be active in every living circulation in order to lift it out of gravity. The etheric or formative-force body calls substances into life; in doing so, it lifts the biological process out of gravity, out of the terrestrial field of forces, and opens it to cosmic influences. The sucking tendency of the grips supports the action of the etheric body. Finally, we should like to mention the introduction of the *lemniscate* and its variations, which has proved to be an especially effective form of motion for the harmonizing and gathering of biological force activities.

In the courses for beginners the fundamental forms are learned, only later a freer manipulation of these forms can be acquired. Everything connected with healing is much more closely connected with the artistic element than with technique. Yet at the basis of every art there must lie an exact technique.

14.

HARMONY AND DISHARMONY OF THE MEMBERS OF MAN'S BEING

The spiritual-scientific image of man leads to a *new conception of health and illness*. We have already pointed to the fact that the harmonious interplay of the members of man's being, in the sense of the threefold membering of the functional organism, appears as health. Illness appears when the activities of the members of man's being are shifted and encroach upon regions which cannot bear their way of action. This is a description of the phenomenon, but it says nothing about the causes for the shift.

From the observation of the threefold organism, whole categories of disease tendencies can easily be deciphered if one of the functional regions pushes its activity into another.

The upper pole, the nerve-sense system, is characterized by breaking down processes accompanying the waking 'day processes.' Formation, tendency toward mineralization, phenomena of condensation, that is materialization, predominate here, connected with the slowing down of the life processes and the phenomena of cold, of low temperature. Paracelsus summed up these processes, as already mentioned, in the concept *'Sal processes.'* If these forces penetrate into the rhythmical system, if they increase, there arise stoppages and disturbances of the rhythmical activities in the whole organism. Finally, pathological changes occur in the direction indicated. Deposits of various kinds arise, from the finest to the coarsest *sclerotic tendencies*, accompanied by spasms and cramps of every degree in the organs of the rhythmical system, such as the vascular and respiratory systems, up to all stages of coronary heart disease. Rudolf Steiner describes the formation of a tumor as a *displaced formation of a sense organ*. In the metabolic sphere the formative, organizing higher members of man's being must not release themselves from the physical as happens in the nerve-sense system. If they do so, a region arises which can proliferate. The Sal formation, which is a normal, healthy process in the nerve-sense sphere, can push through the rhythmical system right into the metabolic system and there it becomes a process of disease. It can easily be seen that our civilization, with its increased use of the nerve-sense system through overintellectualization, aids this kind of illness.

On the other hand, if the warmth-producing, loosening forces of the metabolic pole, which Paracelsus calls the *'Sulphur-processes,'* appear in the foreground, flooding their shores, all kinds of *inflammatory phenomena*, accompanied by liquefactions, melting down, warmth formation, etc., occur. The ancient physicians still valued fever and pus formation as companions in battle against advancing processes of cold and phenomena of condensation. 'Pus bonum et laudabile,' laudable pus, is a phrase that reaches out to us from the past.

In fever, the individuality pushes deeper into the body, it exerts itself more strongly in order to get the better of a hardening disease, the preponderance of the nerve-sense pole. Fever should be fought against only if the pendulum swings too far to the side of the sulphuric forces. In pneumonia, for instance, fever signifies self-help for overcoming the densificaiton of the lungs. The opposite is the case in tuberculosis, when the loosening forces push up from metabolism too violently into the lungs and destroy the tissue. The lack of the power of materialization leads here distinctly to the disappearance of body substances.

The nerve-sense pole slows down, the metabolic pole accelerates the processes; therefore it is the febrile attacks that are acute. Both poles are connected with each other by a certain elastic tension. They stimulate each other's activity. Rhythm, as a balancing process, must lie between the two. Only when the inner *Mercury* has established equilibrium between the two poles can recovery occur. Every human being has an individual interplay of the members of his being and, therefore, also his individual health as well as his individual tendency toward illness.

Schematic abstraction in the art of healing always misses reality. It needs earnest study and practical experience to be able to recognize the special situation of the individual man, even if at first only in rough outline.

In his lecture of February 11, 1923, *The Invisible Man Within Us*,* Rudolf Steiner describes as an example the process of a splinter pushed into the body. Two things may happen. The irritation of the foreign body calls up both poles, the force of inflammation and the condensing force of form. If the splinter is finally encapsulated then the condensing mineralizing force of the upper man has been victorious. If the splinter festers, the loosening forces of the metabolic pole preponderates. When the splinter is removed or has grown into the flesh, equilibrium is restored. The course of many a disease shows an oscillation between the two poles of forces; first there is an inflammatory and then a degenerative sclerotic state in one and the same illness or a progression in recurrences. *Arthritis* is a living example of this, also *multiple sclerosis*; in brief, everything that takes it course in recurrences.

The middle system always tries to create a balance. It consists of breathing and circulation. *Respiration* is, as it were, the finger which the breaking-down forces extend into the centre; and again expressed pictorially, metabolism extends *circulation* upward as its finger. Respiration is a gently breaking-down process, the pulse in circulation is a gently upbuilding process. This fact may at first cause surprise. It may easily be understood that violent breathing causes a breaking down, a consuming; it is less known that the pulse contains an upbuilding element. Pulsating fluids are more

---

*   Rudolf Steiner, *The Invisible Man Within Us*, Mercury Press, New York, 1978.

living than stationary fluids. Pulsating springs show gently upbuilding, imponderable healing forces, stimulating regeneration. *Rhythmical pulsation* is equal to a gentle etherization. It is the same process that underlies the potentizing of a remedy in the fluid medium. The 'potency' is thereby permeated by the effects of formative forces that gradually take the place of the purely physical effects of substances. With this is connected the fact that regulated rivers in a bed of concrete have dead water without self-purifying forces and that rivers meandering in a lively way with rhythmical changes keep their connection with the cosmic world of formative forces.

Let us return to the human organism. Breath and blood processes, breath and pulse, confront one another in the centre in a cosmic rhythm of one to four. Normally, there are four pulse beats to one breath. Rudolf Steiner points to the fact - as has already been described in the chapter, "Circulation and Heart" - that here *a sun rhythm is implanted into man that is connected with the inmost nature of his entelechy*. I repeat the description because of the great significance of this process. On the average, 72 pulse beats accompany 18 breaths in one minute. We have in one day 18 x 6 x 24 breaths, that is to say, 25,920 breaths. This is the number of years it takes the vernal point to move once through the zodiac. Every year at the vernal equinox, the point of the ecliptic at which the sun rises moves back a certain distance. At the time of Christ this point was in *Aries*; today it is in *Pisces*. This fact is of fundamental significance for the evolution of the human race, because this great course of the sun determines the character of the cultural periods which take their course in a definite sign of the zodiac. Prior to the sign of Aries, the vernal point stood in the sign of *Taurus*. The leading culture of that period was the Egyptian with its bull rituals. Earlier still, the sun rose at the vernal equinox in the sign of *Gemini*. The ancient Persian culture of Zarathustra developed at that time with its mighty conception of the duality of light and darkness, of the archetypal polarity of Good, revered in the sun as Ahura Mazdao, and Evil, perceived in the demon of darkness, Ahriman. The great sun rhythm is the leading one in the evolution of the human race.

Spirit and soul have been 'breathed into us' if we wish to retain the Biblical expression with the sun rhythm. As regards the relationship of four pulse beats to one breath, let us briefly recall that we related the four members of man's being with the four basic numbers and the four elements; then a first light may fall upon this relationship of one to four. I should like to express it carefully; if the *spirit* is to work into the *physical body*, into the element earth, the rhythm must be 1:4, *fire to earth*. In the structure of the rhythmical system itself, on the other hand, there is concealed the central rhythm 2:3, *air to water*, two lobes of the lung on the left side to three lobes of the lung on the right side together with the bronchial ramifications. Likewise we find two valves in relation to three valves in the heart, left and right. This 2:3 would indicate here an especially important relationship between *astral body* and *ether body*, between soul and life, and it is these two that merge in the middle man. It is self-evident that there are still quite different possibilities of elucidating our middle system; what has been described here may suffice. This originally cosmic rhythm is, like everything else, individualized by man, nobody has a completely exact measure, but its shifting always indicates the particular force relationship of the poles.

The following must be added. The soul-spiritual can only dive down into the body because the blood contains iron. *Iron is the metal of respiration*; it is the mighty cosmic substance that can bind the soul-spiritual to the physical-bodily. In this sense it is the metal of incarnation. If it is lacking we become too plant-like, we cannot retain the astral body and the ego.

I here draw attention to the cardinal statement of Spiritual Science; namely, that the spirit must always act through substance if it wants to reveal itself on the physical plane. We only know the complicated world of substances separated form the spiritual as a dead world in itself. We must slowly recognize the substances of which spirit and soul must make use in order to fulfill their tasks in the physical world. The first step toward such knowledge was the insight that the spirit can work directly only through the element fire, the soul through the gaseous, life through the fluid element. Solely the earth element belongs to the dead mineral forces. Iron in the warm blood, in living fire, is the bearer of the movement of breath, it leads the astral body and the ego to submerge into the world of substances of the organism. The ancient Teutons, who experienced in mythological images the working of the soul in the body, saw, for instance, in *Thor with the iron hammer* the same power in the great cosmos that in the microcosm worked in them through the pulsating blood. Thor for them was a spiritual being who worked on the *creation of the ego*.

Blood, therefore, does not only contain metabolic processes, it is through its content of iron a constant source of curative effects. Thus normally the disease-producing breaking-down processes in the nervous system are constantly healed through the equalizing processes of the blood, and illnesses occur only if the latter do not suffice.

We are constantly a patient through the onesided processes of the two poles that have had *to arise through the embodying of our soul and spirit*, and we are at the same time to a certain degree our own doctor, our own Mercury, through the processes of the rhythmical system in the centre.

It is the task of massage, expanded through spiritual- scientific knowledge, to become in its way a helper of this inner Mercury if his forces do not suffice. Every remedy is limited to a certain region; and massage is no cure-all. *In a regulating fashion* it acts chiefly *upon the rhythmical activities* and from there it is able to strengthen or soothe the one or the other pole through the quality of its grips and the place of application. Here we have only characterized the basic thought. In the further elaboration many problems will arise when we go into the details. This can, however, only be done against the background of the *spiritual-scientific image of man*. The masseur must penetrate deeper and deeper into the observation of the phenomena the patient presents. The new image of man facilitates the matter insofar as it comes closer to the artistic observation of the world in its imagery. The transition from the science of healing to the art of healing can only result through practice. In contrast to a mechanical observation that, according to the pattern of our mechanical world order, believes to see in man a badly or well-functioning factory, the new path, considering the higher principles of life, soul, and spirit, is much more difficult and demands serious study. It lifts the profession into an entirely new and responsible sphere. It is self-evident that the masseur acts only by prescription of the physician, but the way he acts must not be an applied technique, a fixed course of action, but an individual meaningful curative treatment, the scope of which will be dealt with in the subsequent chapters.

15.

THE LAW OF POLARITY IN MASSAGE

In order to make clear the relationships in massage, Rudolf Steiner, in his lectures to physicians, again proceeds from the observation of the two poles by observing as an example the contrast between brain and spleen. The brain is the center of the *conscious life of thought*. The spleen, however, this sponge of blood, is designated as the *center of the unconscious states of willing*. On these facts Rudolf Steiner founds the nature of massage. A second time he describes the same from a somewhat different point of view. I herewith quote both passages.

(From lecture XVI in *Spiritual Science and Medicine*, April 5, 1920):*

"All those processes in the organism whose nature is such that their physical occurrences are accompanied by the higher processes of consciousness, especially by the conceptual processes, are toxic activities in the organism. This must not be overlooked. The organism poisons itself continually precisely through its conceptual activity, and counteracts these toxic conditions continually through the operation of the unconscious will. The center for these conditions of the unconscious will is the spleen. If we stimulate the spleen and imbue it with a certain awareness, by means of massage, we take action against the powerful toxic effects caused by our higher consciousness. And this massage may be applied not only externally but from within as well. You may dispute the term massage in this connection, but you will understand what I mean. . . . Do not confine your intake of food to the chief meals of the day, but rather eat as little as you can at those meals, and take other nourishment in between meals; spread out your consumption of food, so that you eat a little at a time but frequently, at short intervals. The abnormal consciousness of the spleen can be influenced in this way. For to eat a little and often is essentially an internal massage of the spleen, which considerably alters the activity of that organ. Of course, there is a "but;" all that concerns the organic processes under discussion has its "buts." In our age of haste and hurry in which almost everyone is caught up in some exhausting external activity, the spleen and its functions are extraordinarily liable to impairment through this ceaseless round of work. Mankind does not follow the example of certain animals who keep themselves sound and "fit" by lying down to rest

---

*   Rudolf Steiner Press, London, 1975.

after food, so that digestive processes are not disturbed by external activity. These animals are really taking care of their spleen. Man does not take care of his spleen if occupied in some hurried activity at the expense of nervous energy. And therefore the splenetic function in the whole of modern civilized peoples gradually becomes thoroughly abnormal, so that especial significance attaches to its relief and recovery through the sort of remedies I have just indicated.

"Such delicate processes as massage of the spleen, whether external or internal, draw attention to the relationship between those organs of mankind which transmit the unconscious experience, and the other human organs which transmit conscious experiences. They illuminate the whole *significance of massage*. Massage has a certain definite significance and under some circumstances a powerful remedial effect, but above all it influences and regulates *rhythm in man*. The regulation of human rhythmic processes is the main office of massage. And to massage successfully, one must know the human organism well. You will find the way if you consider the following: Think for a moment of the immense difference between *arms and legs* in the human frame, as distinct from the animal. The arms of man, which are liberated from the oppression of weight and can move freely, have their astral body far less closely bound to the physical than in the case of the feet. To the feet the astral body is closely bound. In fact we may say that in the case of the arms the astral body acts from without and inwards through the skin, enveloping arms and hands and working centripetally. In the legs and feet the will works through the astral body very strongly in a centrifugal direction, radiating powerfully outwards, from within. Therefore, if massage is applied to the legs and feet in man, the process is essentially different from that of massage applied to the hands and arms. If the *arms* are treated by massage, the astral element is drawn from outside inwards, and the arms become very much more instruments of the will than they would otherwise be. Through this there is a regulative effect on internal metabolism, especially on that part of the metabolic process taking place between intestine and blood vessels. In short, massage of the upper limbs acts to a great extent on the *formation of the blood*. If, on the other hand, the *feet and legs* are massaged, the physical element is transmuted rather into something of a conceptual nature and a regulative action follows on the metabolism that is concerned with processes of evacuation and excretion. The extreme complexity of the human organism is most clearly revealed in these indirect and secondary effects of massage, whether starting from the arms and mainly affecting the upbuilding internal processes of metabolism, or starting from the legs and feet and affecting the disintegrating processes of metabolism. If you investigate rationally, you will indeed find that every bodily region and part has a certain connection with other regions and parts, and that the efficacy of massage depends on an adequate insight into these interrelationships. *Massage of the lower body* will always be of benefit even to the *function of breathing*, a circumstance of special interest. And in fact, the farther we go from above downwards, we find that the organs above the center benefit progressively. For example, massage directly below the cardiac region influences respiration; if we go farther down, the organs of the throat are influenced. It is a reversed process; the farther we descend from the center, in massage of the trunk, the greater the effect on the upper organs. And, strangely enough, massage treatment of the arms is much helped by massage of the uppermost region of the trunk. These facts illustrate the interlocking of the individual regions and limbs of the human body."

From *Physiology and Therapeutics*, lecture of October 9, 1920*:

"Let us take examples from a field that can lead us at the same time into the entire connection of spirit and soul with the physical. What is imparted in human life through the nerve-sense system signifies the conscious life of man from awaking to going to sleep. We may say: the head system is the expression of the conscious life of man. The metabolic system, however, is not in the same sense the expression for man's conscious life. We go through the world, as it were, with conscious head yet with unconscious limbs. These limbs become conscious only if they are touched or wounded in some way. In the waking state, consciousness is the normal state for the head and nerve system, unconsciousness for the opposite system.

It is possible, however, artificially to produce in man a kind of consciousness for the metabolic-limb system. This happens for instance through massage. It consists in making conscious through external means what otherwise remains unconscious. One can try through massage to improve the connection of spirit and soul with the physical body. Let us assume a human being is organized unhealthily through the fact that he has too little inclination to drive his spirit and soul completely into his metabolic-limb system. Then the physical element of this metabolic-limb system is supported by massage, by lifting the spiritual into the state of consciousness, calling forth a stronger permeation of the physical element with spirit and soul. And if one understands the activity of this metabolic-limb system, if one knows, for instance, that the spirit and soul element that

---

* Rudolf Steiner, *Physiology and Therapeutics*, Mercury Press, Spring Valley, 1986.

pulsates in the arms and hands continues on and controls the inner metabolism of man, then one also knows the significance of producing a partial consciousness in the arms and hands through massage. It signifies a furtherance of the spirit-soul element in the metabolic system, in that metabolic system that produces in man an inward up-building process effecting digestion which absorbs substance.

Thus we may say: If we find that the human being suffers inwardly organically from metabolic disturbances which are caused by the fact that his food does not properly join with the body or that digestion of his food in the up-building process does not properly take place, in other words, that metabolism moving inward is not in order, then in certain cases of course we must know the details in order to view this in the right way the massage of arms and hands may be helpful. This rests upon the fact that spirit and soul are supported in their effect through the degree of consciousness produced through massage. If we massage legs and feet something different occurs. What as spirit and soul permeates legs and feet has an organic connection with the processes of secretion. Therefore, if digestion is not in order in regard to the proper performance of the processes of secretion, under certain circumstances massage of the legs and feet may be helpful."

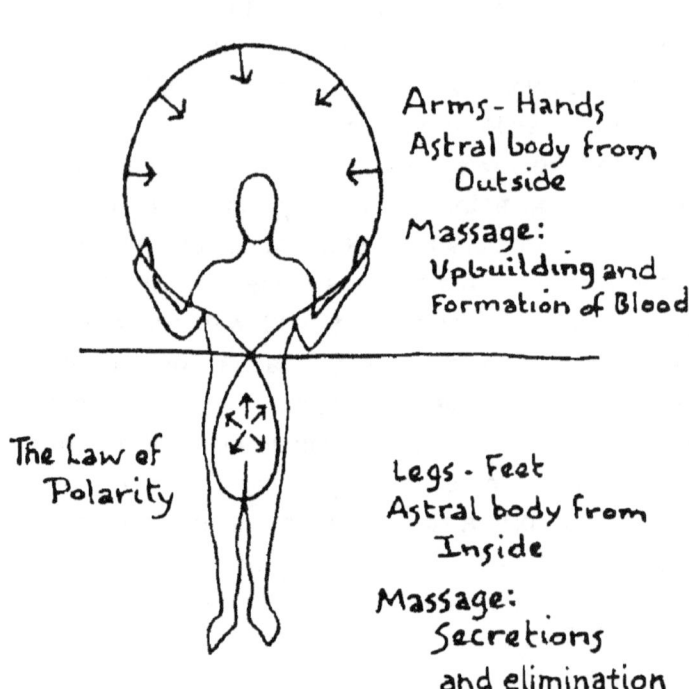

These are the only passages in which Rudolf Steiner speaks about the nature of massage. They contain, if observed more closely, everything that can lead to a completely new departure in this domain. I am fully conscious of the fact that the content of this book presents merely a beginning of what Rudolf Steiner expected as an elucidation of this domain with spiritual-scientific thoughts, for he once stated that in many cases proper massage might replace the knife of the surgeon. We can anticipate this if we grasp the fact that here we have an instrument in our hand, literally in our hand, that can direct the activity of the astral body through binding and releasing in the most differentiated manner. In the second paragraph of this quotation we find the earnest sentence: 'To massage successfully, one must know the human organism well.' Here knowledge is referred to that comprises the activity of the higher members of man's being, and it becomes clear that the body has always to be considered as a totality. The whole participates in every change and the effects are transmitted according to the laws of the various members of man's being. Here, at the outset, the *law of polarity of the astral body* is applied. This becomes comprehensible from what has been described so far. Completely new, however, is the fact that the applications for arms and legs have such different effects upon the metabolism. We have to add, concerning the fact that massage of the lower man affects elimination, that the functioning of the secreting glands is a kind of submerged motion of breathing, a binding and releasing of the astral body from the physical-etheric. If the astral body acts in an organizing way from inside, submerged below the level of the etheric body, secretion is built up; this corresponds to the situation of the members of man's being in the region of the up-building metabolism. If the astral body loosens itself partially, secretions are eliminated, abandoned; this corresponds to the situation of the members of man's being in the upper man. This becomes clear through the fact that the secretions are very important for the formation of consciousness and, closely observed, are always accompanied by a brightening of consciousness.

Upbuilding of Secretion

Astral Body

Secretion

Man is more easily conscious of the opposite; namely, *dullness through deficient activity of the secreting glands* which, in certain illnesses, may lead to a darkening of consciousness, even loss of consciousness if it is a case of vital secretions.

In order to avoid misunderstandings I should like to emphasize the fact that one always massages the physical body, but one knows it to be permeated and differentiated by the spiritual-soul element and the life processes. To make conscious the various bodily parts through the process of massage stimulates various activities of this spiritual-soul element in the body. The body alone would only be a corpse if this interplay of its higher members did not pulsate through it.

Nobody needs to believe the results of Spiritual Science, but testing them in actuality verifies them step by step.

16.

THE QUALITIES OF GRIP

If we become conscious of the fact that in massage we must take hold of the bodily processes from the outside in the same way that man actively does from the inside, it is self-evident that the nature of the grips must lie in the interplay of the four elements. The elements in the Aristotelian sense, fire, air, and water, form the bridge for the intervention of the higher members of man's being, *fire* for the *spiritual-egohood*, *air* for the *soul-astral member*, *water* for the *living-etheric member*. Observation of nature thereby becomes an instructor. Naturally, this can only be a suggestion, since the human organism is a microcosm drawn together into the narrowest space. Nevertheless, the development of a *nature sense* is recommended, to see how air and water treat one another. How the wind tosses up the waves, how vortices are formed, how the streams in the living water are never a straight line, but are gently meandering, how everything breathes, how it is possible that a warm stream flows in the cold ocean, and so on. And above everything else there is the sublime archetypal image of all motion, the exalted loops and circles carried out above us by the astra, the stars. All this should form the background and awaken the soul of the therapist to the true forces of healing which stream to the earth from the cosmos. For the rhythms of the universe, placed between the celestial heights and the depths of the earth, are, also in the cosmos, the principle creating equilibrium between the great polarities. *The Universe, too, is an organism* and not a mechanism. The bodily processes must never be drawn into the field of mechanical motion that is derived from technical instruments. *The earth's field of forces hardens and makes them too physical.* Already at the beginning we mentioned that the five fundamental grips of Swedish Massage were the starting point of our work. We shall characterize them in the following paragraphs.

Stroking (Effleurage)

Stroking contains above all directive forces for the fluid man. The introductory effleurage does not only exist for the spreading of the carrying substance but it is carried out according to certain *guide-lines* which as regards the extremities usually follow the muscles, indeed, even the artistic sculpture of the human body, stimulating the streaming of circulation in the direction of the heart. The good and warm contact of the palm of the hand is important in this procedure. The stroke is light but has to have a good contact. The hand ought to have as little of its own weight as a boat in the water, but it must dip into the stream to the degree that it can drive a gentle bow-wave in front of it, pictorially speaking. A few strokes suffice for stimulation.

Stroking includes the warming *double circles* and, especially, the *lemniscate* that with its metamorphoses is used in various ways. Proceeding from the warmth organism, we include in such strokings larger regions, especially in the back and the joints. This stroke has special significance in rehabilitating sick arms and other parts that have functionally fallen out of the general life stream; in short, to smooth the way for the unifying intervention of the ego. In a later chapter we shall see that the lemniscate is of decisive effect in the regions which serve the ego activity.

Stroking must show still another quality, it must breathe; that is to say, the gentle pressure must not be a continuous one but it must increase and decrease. All these qualities can best be understood from the artistic aspect. The stroke then becomes *musical or colorful*.

It is of special importance that the movement must never contain the so-called 'swing.' Every movement must be under the complete and conscious control of the masseur. The impulse of movement must always be thoughtful. Swing is an expression of the astral body alone. If the ego enters in, the accelerated, seemingly swinging movement is controlled at once. This holds good especially for the movements that end the massage.

Kneading (Petrissage)

Whereas stroking is a breathing movement on the surface, kneading is a deeper reaching rhythmical pulsation. Kneading is a *circulating movement in loops*; its true archetype is the movement of the loops of the planetary orbits. The tissue is touched and sucked up with the full middle hand and then relased again, followed by the next grip. The hand moves constantly on a circle that rolls like a little wheel on the tissue. Kneading may be compared to a cresting, rolling wave.

Round Kneading   Cresting Wave

The wave may be varied in all directions, it is simply a question of skill. Its basic character of a sucking heaving must, however, be retained, even if there is only room for two fingers.

The two-hand kneading always takes place with a shifting of the phases, the impulse must never push simultaneously into both hands of the masseur, both hands must never suck at the same time, but successively. Thereby a rhythm arises which resembles the heart rhythm. A good and deep kneading equals the formation of a kind of *peripheral heart activity* for the capillary region of skin, subcutaneous cellular tissue and musculature. The motion then moves on two circles which penetrate each other. This also is a fundamental principle which may be individually transformed in all directions.

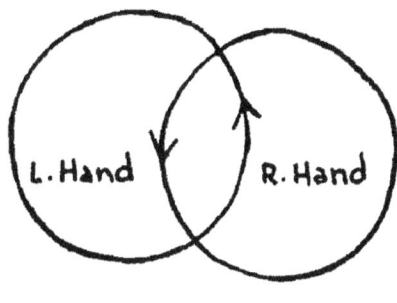

Two-Hand Kneading

The motion is two circles that run after one another (shifting of the phases) and thereby interpenetrate each other in counter-movement.

Airy Kneading ("Walken")

This is a kind of airy, strongly sucking, kneading, with both hands, whereby one tries, in the case of a limb, to loosen the whole muscle from the bone. It is only applied on the extremities and in a slightly changed form on the abdomen. It is necessary that the motion is harmoniously brought to rest and the tissue is not simply dropped. To use an expression of musical sensitivity: one has to end with a final chord. This may be a short stroke or any slow, emphasized form.

Friction

Through the way they reach into the depths and through their rubbing character, frictions serve especially in the production of breaking down processes which are connected with a stronger consciousness. They have their model in the whirlwind that arises between air and water, or air and air of varying temperatures. A friction is like a *small spiral movement into the depths* and a returning upward. Frictions above the colon make this especially clear. There one has no bony base and really reaches as though in a funnel into the depths. *Frictions awaken the breaking down astral body.* They are useful wherever tissue hypertrophy and nodules show a pathological accumulation of deposited substances, preferably near the joints or around certain nerve points. There exists a special method, the *nerve point massage of Professor Cornelius*, which consists solely in frictions of the nerve points. Here the attention is directed to the elastic tension between nerve pole and blood pole. Friction causes a stimulus in the nervous system; in the counter thrust of the blood pole loosening forces can develop, restoring the healthy relationship of the members of man's being. We can compare the effect of this with short applications of cold which are and have to be followed by the healing warming from the side of the blood, otherwise the application is not wholesome. In states of exhaustion with deficiency in reaction great care has to be taken. Frictions whose fundamental character has been described can take on forms that are not circular. Yet the massage movement must always remain *simple and in harmony with the body*. It must never be an intellectually thought-out movement that is applied to the body from outside. A good masseur moves what lies below the skin, he inserts himself into the functions of the tissue. External movements will have little effect. Worse still is the overpowering of the tissue. Here, what the Greeks understood by virtue becomes visible once more; namely, the balance between too little and too much.

Tapotement, Percussion

Percussion is carried out with the fingers held fanwise, successively tapping, either on one point or spread out; it must be, above all, *light and springy*. This has a stimulating effect upon the astral body. Applied on the back, it deepens breathing and loosens mucus. It may also be applied to completely relaxed large muscles and is comparable to a refreshing rain shower.

Vibration

Vibrations also serve the loosening of the cramped astral body in asthma and other bronchial obstructions with phlegm. They may also be used on the abdomen in chronic constipation. The two last kinds of grip belong to the manipulations not springing from the basic form. Gentle shaking, slight stretching and similar special grips belong to this category that is known in almost every technique of massage.

On the whole the practice of decades has shown that *having mastered these grip qualities no additional manipulations are needed*. If one knows the organism well, one can produce with these grips all the effects lying in the domain of this method of healing.

Through knowledge of the polar activity of the astral body the *indications* for massage are considerably *enlarged*. To the general *regulation of the rhythmical activities* and the *stimulation of the building up and elimination processes* in the widest sense there must be added the whole domain of the *diversion massages* in which one works on the opposite side of the disease process in order to divert the activity of the astral body which at a certain place is perhaps too violent and causes congestion, even inflammation. These conditions will be dealt with separately in the description of individual procedures of treatment.

17.

THE USE AND QUALITY OF OILS IN RHYTHMICAL MASSAGE

To have a *biological lubricant* is not the only reason for using oil in Rhythmical Massage, but in most treatments the physician will prescribe oil that contains a *special curative substance*.

In order to visualize the qualities of the ethereal as well as the fatty oils I refer to the descriptions by Rudolf Hauschka in his book, *The Nature of Substance*, where the oils are dealt with in connection with the entire field of plant substances. There it becomes evident that the *oil formation process* is the *final and highest synthesis* in the seed formation whereby the plant reaches its crowning process.

Above the plant: Fragrance, Oil, Honey, Curative Substances, Colour
Within the plant: Sugar ↑ Starch ↓ Cellulose
Below the plant: Coal Tar, Saccharine, Mineral Oil, Tar Colour, Aspirin, Thalidomide, etc., Synthetic Perfume

In this connection Rudolf Hauschka describes the *ethereal oils* as pre-stages, as *childhood of the genuine oils*. The drawings from the book, *The Nature of Substance*, (page 93 and below), elucidate the series of processes in the plant.

The first drawing shows the stream of substance formation in the plant between cosmos and earth. At the top are the substances it develops in the blossom through the interplay with the cosmic forces. And in the mirrored image of it we find what the human intellect is able to develop from the coal tar. Above, the laws of life hold sway: below, the laws of atomic and molecular chemistry.

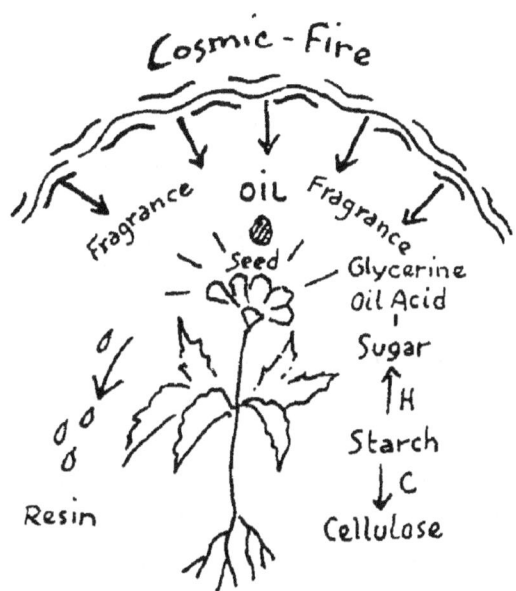

The second drawing elucidates especially the origin of oil. Oil can be split into two parts if we destroy it through alkalis; namely, into oil or fatty acid and a component resembling alcohol, glycerine. The share of acid in the plant is to be found in the swelling seed-bud. These plant acids in the ovary of the plant, Rudolf Hauschka calls the vessel 'into which is received the being of fragrance radiated back from the periphery of the cosmos. The fire force of this being warms through and permeates the arising structure; as an expression of their collaboration there comes into being before us the substance of oil. In this sense oil is to be called *the perfect plant substance.*' For this very reason, oil was always a ritual substance which, originating in the spirit-bearing cosmic fire, anointed the heads of priests and kings in their high offices, or which as last anointing accompanied the return into the spiritual world.

Just as salt is composed of acid and alkali, so oil is composed of *plant acid and glycerine*. It is a higher biological synthesis. Formed by cosmic warmth, these *oils and resins keep the plant united with its prototype*. Through their connection with fire, they carry the spiritual prototype through the seed state over into the future development and thus form the warranty for a new germinal development of the same plant shape.

In general, the fatty oils have the following effect upon the skin: they keep together our total being within the organism and thereby weaken the hardening and isolating earth forces, and above all the subsensory forces of the electro-magnetic field. Just as we, through the ego, consolidate and strengthen our personality of spirit and soul, so oil, through the *consolidation of the warmth organism* assists the ego in a better and more orderly intervention in the biological processes.

Considering the fatty oils as a perfect substance resting in itself, we see the *ethereal oils*, through *enrichment with hydrogen*, on the side of evaporation. Their fragrance is only pleasant in dilution. The resins, on the other hand, have been made more earthly through *enrichment with oxygen*. They give their fire nature a more inward character. Only if they are burnt do they reveal their fragrance and release their 'spirit' (as these volatile substances have characteristically been called when they become free through the heating of resins). Thus resin of turpentine when heated releases first the volatile spirit of turpentine, then the heavier oil of turpentine, and as a residue there remains colophony, a waxlike substance. Frankincense is another resin. If it is lighted it symbolizes, in the language of the ritual, the feeling of devotion streaming from the human breast and revering the divinity. The resins contain latent forces that rest enclosed within them and which fire releases.

In the production of massage oils the fatty oil is used as a basis and according to our choice ethereal oils and other remedial substances are added. If we wish to relate the plant processes to man, the plant must be reversed. Its *root processes* with the salts act upon the head region with its sal-processes, upon the formative nerve-sense processes. The *leaves* are related to respiration and circulation in the sphere of Mercurial processes. The *blossom* substances are related to the sulphuric metabolic region. The *seed*, finally, acts chiefly upon the heart where everything is again comprised as in the seed.

These relationships are valid in general. Yet the plant itself shifts these processes in its own structure according to its genus, and there are endless variations and particularities.

If the physician does not prescribe differently, one uses an oil that stimulates the *skin functions* in general. The *Wala-Heilmittel Laboratorium* (Laboratory for Wala Remedies) in Eckwälden has an oil production program suited to these treatments whereby through application of warmth rhythms during extraction the relationship to the deeper qualities of the oil is specially emphasized. Naturally, every other good oil may be used.

The oil must be used sparingly in order to prevent the slipping off of the massage grips through too thick an oil layer and to bring about a depth effect through really good contact. Superfluous oil must always be wiped off, otherwise it leaves behind a feeling of cold. There exist great differences in regard to the capacity of resorption of the oil which are based upon the constitution of the patient. Here experience must decide.

Mineral oils or talcum are never used in the rhythmical treatments.

18.

RHYTHM

Evolution in time is carried by numerous rhythms; hours, days, weeks, years flow along and still greater rhythms are caused by ever-changing relationships of sun, moon and stars to one another, by the fact that they move.

Thus all life in time is carried by rhythms. Rudolf Steiner's term for the life functions of man is ether organism or formative force body. This is a first supersensible body. We can designate it as our time body. Time rules in it. It has its cosmic counterpart in the etheric world of the formative forces of the cosmos. This world of rhythms is a *mediator world*. It mediates the soul-spiritual forces to the earthly bodily element. The path from the spiritual into the manifestation of the bodily always leads through a rhythm, and also the path of the spiritualization of earthly substance leads through rhythms. Between the physical world and the soul-spiritual world there is the world of life permeated by rhythms.

This great truth shines through Goethe's marvellous lines spoken by the Spirit of the Earth to Faust:

> In the tides of life, in action's storm
> Up and down I weave,
> To and fro weave free,
> Birth and the grave,
> An infinite sea,
> A varied weaving,
> A radiant living,
> Thus at Time's humming loom it's my hand that prepares
> The robe ever living the Deity wears.

(translated by George Madison Priest)

All creation, everything we see, has condensed out of life rhythms. Mineral substances are the final sediment of creation and have fallen out of life. Only rhythmical processes, that man can learn from the Cosmos, are able to bring the earth substances close again to their spiritualization. And it is the immortal merit of Hahnemann to have made the first step upon this path to the future with his concept of 'potentization.' A potency is a latent force that is released through a rhythmical process, it is a substance lifted toward the life sphere. Today we are only at the beginning of research in this new world of formative forces, but with this research into the significance of rhythm we stand before the portal of a new age and a new science.*

From all this it becomes clear that rhythm belongs to the concept of life. Everybody knows that an activity carried out rhythmically needs less strength. There is a great difference between rhythm and beat. *Rhythm belongs to the world of life, beat to the mechanical, dead world*. Everybody has experienced that it does not tire him to watch the rhythmical play of waves on the shore, but he could hardly stand it for five minutes to watch the beat-like movement of a machine without yawning.

The world of rhythms is inexhaustible. A rhythm always creates the balance between two worlds, two polarities. Let us take our own heart rhythm with systole and diastole: death and life are entwined in it. We live to the extent that we can wrest life from death. The rhythms of poetry with short and long meter tear away language from the paralyzing everyday earth domain and bestow a higher life upon it.

Thus, is it not evident that in the science of healing rhythm is quite especially cultivated? This does not mean that in massage special rhythms are applied, such as the iambic or trochaic rhythm of poetry, but it means that in general one works musically, rhythmically. This rhythm, however, must not be intellectually thought out and applied from outside, but it must be found through entering with one's feeling into the situation, and it will always be akin to the heart rhythm, sometimes slow, sometimes faster as needed in the individual case. Our age has great difficulty in paying sufficient attention to the importance of rhythm. It would never have been necessary to recommend rhythm to a Greek. In sensing his own life rhythms he would quite naturally have carried out his actions rhythmically. In massage, the transitions, the transformations of the grips into one another are of special importance, forming the treatment into a therapeutic organism. The sequence of definite grips alone does not constitute the curative element just as little as the chemical consistency of a substance alone constitutes the remedy. It needs the re-enlivening of the dead substance or the dead technique through man. We practise the art of healing insofar as we wrest the living from dead knowledge and make healing into an individual creative deed. This means that *the substance or the remedy*, whatever it may be, must be *humanized*. An unfortunate indifference in regard to man has entered our medical science. There is a tendency to regard the organism as a machine although a biological one that can be steered and for which there are spare parts. I here express myself drastically on purpose because our brilliant technology deceives us in many respects.

Rhythmical Massage means to shape one's kneadings and strokings in movements of a tempo and continuity in tune with the human being, that is musically.

---

*   Rudolf Hauschka, *Nature of Substance*, Rudolf Steiner Press.

In *music* we possess an *earthly reflection of cosmic forces of order*. Plato speaks of the harmony of the spheres, Goethe still speaks of the sounding orbit of the sun. This musical force of order radiates right down into matter and can be recognized in the laws of chemistry. *Rudolf Hauschka* devotes a whole chapter in his book *Heilmittellehre* to the theme, 'Music in Matter.' If we thus give to our movements a musical character and do not add our grips but *compose* them into a totality, pictorially speaking, then we have immersed the treatment into an atmosphere serving life. But all these indications must not lead to applying them playfully. We only want to show how the divine work of art of man's physical body can be understood much better and deeper through an artistic consideration that through a purely scientific evaluation according to measure, number, and weight. Likewise, it would be trivial and a grave misunderstanding were we to apply this music externally.

All these facts are nothing new for many people; they use them instinctively. But these good qualities may soon be lost if they are not taken hold of consciously by a new spiritual insight and justified in accordance with the need for knowledge of our time.

The fact that the *application of rhythms* has already entered the practice of the *production of remedies* is corroborated by Dr. Rudolf Hauschka's procedure in the conservation of living plant juices. Here the living connections between substances are saved from decay through the use of rhythms, not by killing of the lower bacterial life but by preservation of the higher life connections. Details may be found in Rudolf Hauschka's book *Heilmittellehre* in the chapter about "New Paths in the Production of Remedies."

Rudolf Steiner has pointed out certain special rhythms and cyclic courses. We have already mentioned the great rhythm of 25,920 breaths per day and the corresponding pulse beats.

Also the members of our being, the ego or the spirit, the astral body or the soul, the etheric body or the living formative forces, have their own rhythms, their cyclic periods taking place in them, and repeating themselves. Thus *the ego has a rhythm of 24 hours*; that is, of a day. The ego is the principle set above all polarities: day and night, light and darkness, heaven and earth, etc. This would signify that those processes which are chiefly subject to the ego activity show a 24 hour rhythm. To this belong the day rhythms of many glandular secretions with a morning flood and secretion phase and an evening ebb in the upbuilding and enrichment phase. Dr. Wachsmuth devotes a whole chapter in his book *Earth and Man* to these relationships. The activity of liver and gall is especially controlled by this, as is proved by the already mentioned fact that these processes chiefly underlie the ego activity in metabolism. Included in this are waking and sleeping and many day rhythms of blood circulation, respiration, body temperature. This rhythm reaches up into the behaviour of our spirit and soul with regard to the quite different quality of our efficiency in the morning and in the evening.

Our soul-member, *the astral body, has a rhythm of seven days* which corresponds to its archetype in the seven-membered world of the planets. The astral body, which is excessively active in acute illness, shows itself in the course, for instance, of pneumonia where the crisis occurs on the seventh to ninth day. A finer observation can find the course of other illnesses structured in one week periods, or it can be observed that after a week the soul has reached a certain point of new orientation and that in soul injuries after one or a multiple of weeks balance has been restored if one does not intervene.

Our *life or formative force body has the rhythm of four times seven days*. It is inserted in the body of fluids. Everybody knows that the monthly rhythm of the woman is such a rhythm of twenty-eight days. There are also growth rhythms of twenty-eight days. Rudolf Hauschka was the first to point to these rhythms. Experiments with the growing and decaying of living substances established the fact that the formation of substance reaches its maximum at full moon, its minimum at new moon (*Heilmittellehre*, Chapter IX).

Finally, the *physical body* which, corresponding to the activity of substance, is slow in its motion, needs *one year* to carry out one 'revolution,' that is to say, to come again to the same place in the changes taking place in it. Every physician knows that serious operations, closely observed, need *one year* to be overcome completely. After one year the physical body can newly arrange itself with the other members of man's being; in other words, it can newly insert itself into their activities.

These rhythms were implanted into the members of man's being in times of mankind's evolution long past.

19.

THE LEMNISCATE AND THE PENTAGRAM

As has been described, Rhythmical Massage consists of so-called *fundamental forms* and their *free elaborations*. The fundamental forms are, as it were, the archetypes whose guidelines are derived from the body and which for every bodily region form a particular series of grips only valid for that particular region. Only when the masseur is master of these basic forms can he use them more freely and metamorphose them for a definite case, perhaps joining several forms or inserting special elaborations. Every treatment, however, should always have a basic form as a kind of scaffolding in order to achieve a totality, an organism. This has nothing to do with the length or brevity of the treatment. Even a few orderly grips may be effective for it is a matter of inner discipline.

In the training courses the basic forms are taught first and in the advanced courses the possibilites of variation. Within the forms of motion that first consist of streaming circles and lines, the special form of the lemniscate is above all introduced.

For and understanding of the lemniscate as the motive form assigned to the living world of the sun, I refer to the work of George Adams (*The Plant Between Sun and Earth*) and Rudolf Hauschka (*Heilmittellehre*, Chapter XIV). In the lemniscate the interweaving of cosmic and earthly forces can be expressed. It is thus basic for all physical-etheric life processes, represented in its purest form by the plant which possesses only a life body into which the higher principles act from outside. The two spaces which the lemniscate encloses represent the etheric sun space with forces radiating outward and the earth space radiating inward.

It is not possible to show here in detail the constructions that lead to the drawing shown on the following page. The lemniscate proves to be a curve which represents the harmonious function of equalization between these polarities. It plays a most important part in the organism. It represents the highest principle of the sunlike ego active in warmth and repeats itself constantly in the small and the most minute as the functional curve that in the middle creates the balance between the nerve-sense pole and the metabolic system. I call to mind here the lemniscate between vertebra and rib space which lies at the basis of the entire metamorphosis of the skeleton, or the lemniscate in the heart muscle. *Every breathing motion is a functional lemniscate*.

Thus the *Mercury staff* contains a lemniscate. According to the Greeks, Apollo gave to Mercury the staff of snakes so that he might bind and release, put to sleep and awaken. These are the two directions of motion within the lemniscate; the direction from the sun space to the earth space equals waking up, the direction from the earth space to the sun space equals going to sleep. The Mercury symbol has many interpretations, but one thing is certain: it belongs to the God of the art of healing, since healing consists in the equalizing of the two poles which, acting singly, produce illness. Thus it becomes clear that the lemniscate as a form of motion is employed wherever there is need for a special activity of the ego, of production of warmth, of harmonious connection. Thus it is preferably used on the back, but also on the joints which are places of heightened ego activity like small repetitions of the head formation. Finally, the lemniscate dominates in the embrocation of the organs that need a breathing form of movement which returns into itself.

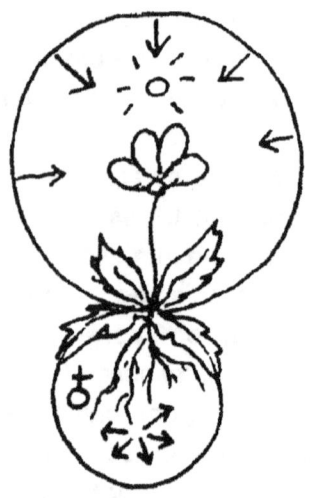

The Plant between Sun and Earth

A second form connected with the sunlike ego of man is the *pentagram* which also in the physical body has an orienting significance. Whereas the lemniscate is the functional curve of harmonious equalization, the pentagram is a mathematical representation of the relationship of the limbs and the head formation to one another. The pentagram, too, signifies the formation of man and was known as such in all the ancient mysteries. The pentagram inscribed in the circle puts the human form into the circle. This human form is streamed through by the etheric body, and the etheric body, lifted through the ego to the level of man, streams in the form of the pentagram.

This movement is carried out in eurythmy by five people moving simultaneously in the form of the pentagram progressivley from point to point. Thereby a *systole* and *diastole* becomes visible in a marvellous way, a contraction and expansion, the primal gesture of the sunlike, breathing formative forces. *A pentagram stream is imprinted*

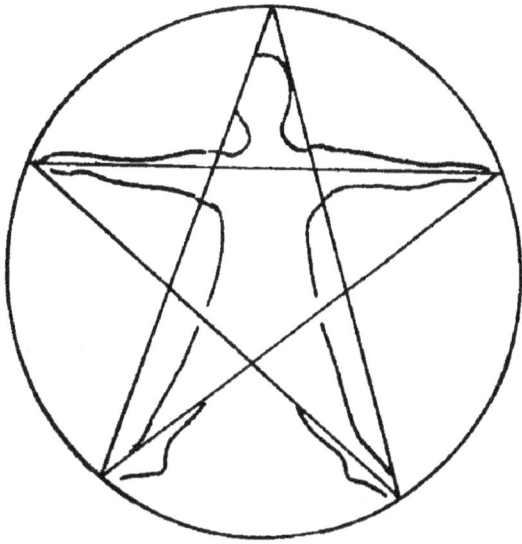

upon the ether body through the ego. Thus in the formation of the limbs man is irradiated with the ego forces, with the spirit. I shall quote here a passage from Rudolf Steiner's *Study of Man** for the teachers of Waldorf schools. 'You must think of the limbs as inserted . . . Spirit is in man's limb system. The body is indicated in the limbs . . . , but also the soul lives in it, and likewise the spirit which basically comprises the whole world.' It is, therefore, not the head that has the relationship to the spirituality of the macrocosm; we close it against the world and have our own thoughts. But the limbs are like radii; through them spirituality radiates into us. Thus the thought is justified that the hands and feet are a special formation of the ego in contrast to all animal formations. Through the extremities we are able to fetch forces for the enlivening of the more central parts which have hardened themselves. The pentagramatic streaming in the ether body can be carefully employed in healing if one is conscious of the fact that one has here to do only with directions of streaming, not with evaluations of quality. With massage one can only smooth the paths of forces. Whether these paths are trodden by the higher essential qualities depends on manifold imponderabilities and one must be able to wait quietly.

*   Rudolf Steiner, *The Study of Man*, Rudolf Steiner Press, London, 1966.

20.

THE BASIC FORMS

The basic forms represent something like the *skeleton of Rhythmical Massage*. Only the main features of the basic forms can be described, since the more precise way of application can only be grasped through visual demonstration. The basic forms are applied in all introductory, generally rhythmical, and harmonizing massages. In the further course of a treatment they will be transformed or enlarged as required. The drawings presented here indicate only the *directions of the treatments* of a few special grips since the quality, especially of the double hand grips, cannot be made visible in a picture. Here we must emphasize that the drawings have value as an *aide memoire* for the masseur, not as teaching material. Yet the character of the massage can to a certain degree be read from them. In regard to the basic forms, we would like to add that they do not represent a dogma *in* any way. They have been *read from the living* and have proved effective. The guiding lines follow in most cases the flowing form of the muscle. There are basic forms for the most important regions of the body and for embrocations of the organs which will be discussed in the next chapter.

Attention will have to be paid to the continuous course of a basic form, letting the whole appear as an organic unity, like a *composition with introduction and final chord*. Effleurage forms the introduction and final, decisive strokes, noticeable for the patient, should form the end of the treatment. All these measures lead from the domain of the merely technically arranged grips into the organically living. A certain *individualization* of the grips will always appear and prevent a deadening dogmatism.

Arm Massage

Duration: 15 to 20 minutes for both arms. Arm and shoulder must be bare. Position: Sitting or in a raised reclining position.

1. Effleurage (stroking). We begin with the extensor aspect from the back of the hand, rhythmically in three parts, increasing and with a good ending on the shoulder in the back. This is followed by the stroke for the flexor aspect from the palm of the hand, also in three parts but decreasing with the final stroke on the pectoralis. The extensor side is repeated.

2. Kneading. First the lower arm, extensor, flexor, extensor, first with one hand, then with both hands. Then the upper arm, in a somewhat different position with elbow support. Deep, soft, pulse-like kneading of the extensor, flexor, and again extensor. If necessary, knead the deltoid muscle separately.

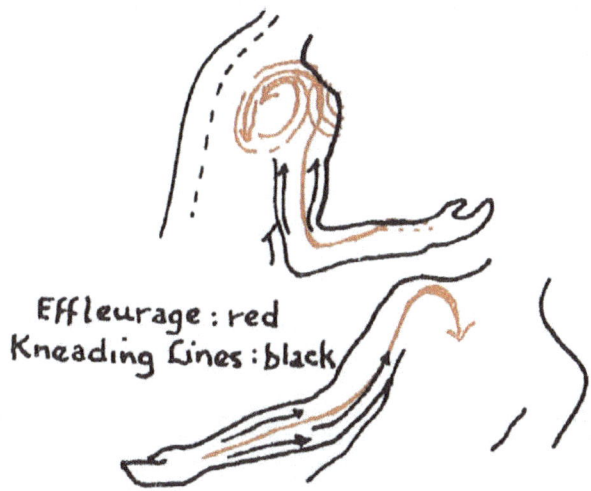

3. Airy Kneading ("Walken"). Airy kneading is applied to the lower arm after the kneading, before the position for the kneading of the upper arm is changed, then airy kneading is applied to the upper arm. The inner hand stops short before the armpit while the outer hand continues on massaging higher up over the deltoid muscle.

4. Moulding circular movements around the joint of the shoulder toward outside with both hands (forming the so-called warmth cap), then leading over along the supraspinatus muscle into a circular movement around the shoulder blade.

Leg Massage from the Front

Whereas the arm can be felt to be a stunted wing (because of the astral body being loosely connected with it) which has only an upper and an under side, and therefore only two guidelines, the leg is completely established in three-dimensional space and has four guide lines.

The treatment of the legs lasts for 20 minutes. The hip must be uncovered. Position: Lying, possibly with slightly raised upper body.

1. Effleurage. With both hands starting at the Achilles tendon, up over the calf with special attention paid to the hollow of the knee, diverting on the thigh into four guiding lines. On the calf all guiding lines converge, above two lines are taken together with both hands until the entire muscle has been well stroked on all sides. Rather firm stroke, but not too long.

2. Kneading. One and two-hand kneading on the calf, starting at the Achilles tendon, then soft and pulse-like kneading upward as with the upper arm with good out stroke in the hollow of the knee. On the thigh all guide lines are kneaded well and rhythmically, beginning with the lower side. For the treatment of the quadriceps, the leg is placed on a light knee roll and then the quadriceps is kneaded with various grips right up into the region of the hip.

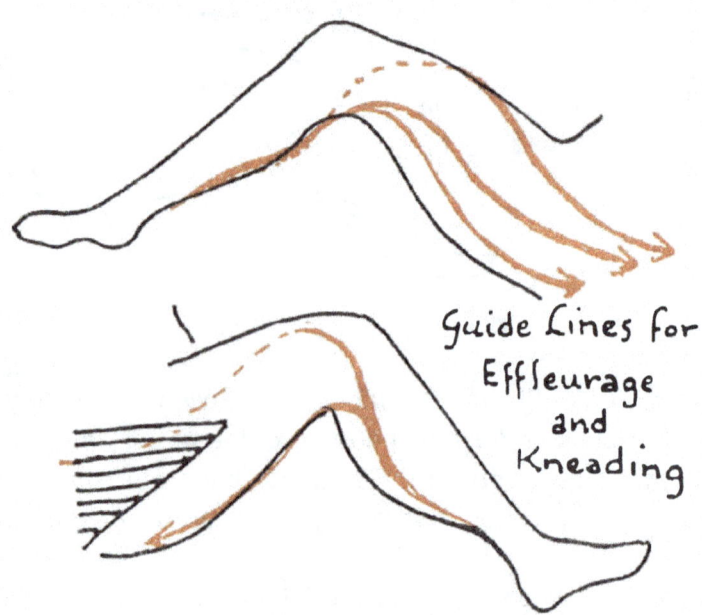

3. Airy Kneading ("Walken"). We try with both hands to free the entire muscle from the bone. Beginning directly above the hollow of the knee, we massage airily up to the trochanter. As in the case of the upper arm the lower hand remains behind, the upper hand, proceeds somewhat higher up. The triangle of the groin (see drawing above) remains untouched during the whole treatment. A few strong out strokes on the guide lines conclude the treatment.

Leg Massage from the Back

Duration: 20 minutes for both legs. Position: lying comfortably on the abdomen with a roll under the feet. Leg and buttocks must be uncovered.

1. Effleurage. With both hands upward from the calf the streams are led past the trochanter and in a curve below the ileac crest toward the lower back, including perhaps, a few circular movements on the buttock. Final stroke on the sacrum.

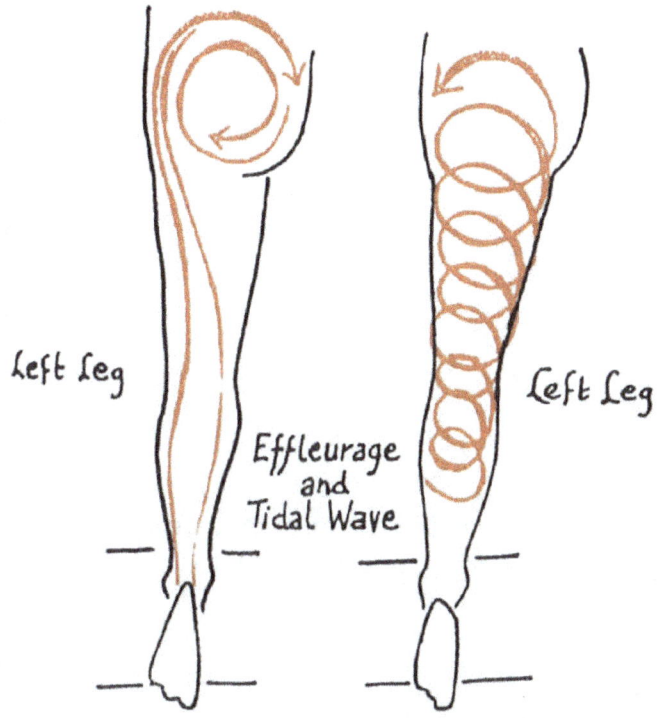

2. Kneading. Covering the upper parts and beginning with the treatment of the region of the Achilles tendon with circular frictions. Then transition to the thorough yet soft and deep kneading of the calf with one and both hands. Kneading of the two flexor groups of the thigh starting below the knee, medially and laterally. The kneading on the outside to be continued on to the buttocks. There circular kneading and final strokes as in the beginning.

3. Airy Kneading ("Walken"). Loosening air kneading on lower leg and thigh. Finally, warming circles form the calf upward like mounting tidal waves. Special attention is paid to the hollow of the knee. If needed, the lower back may be treated in addition in this position.

Massage of the Lower Back

Intensive stroking of the rhombic region and loosening of the entire tissue.

Ray-like treatment through lifting finger kneading. Conclusion with warming lemniscate the loops of which are bent upward.

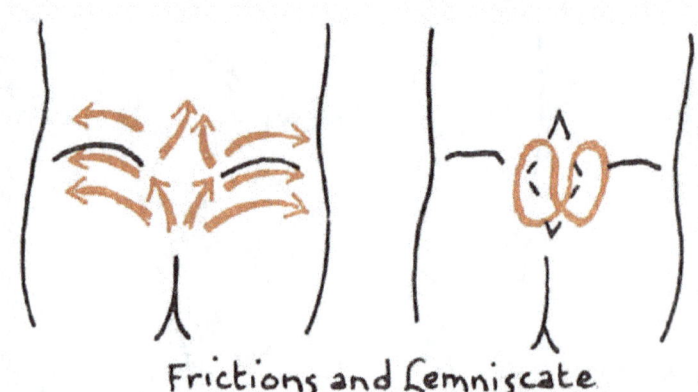

Frictions and Lemniscate

Massage of the Hip

Duration: for both hips 20 to 25 minutes. Position: side position with a pillow against abdomen. The legs are slightly pulled up. Hip and lower back are uncovered.

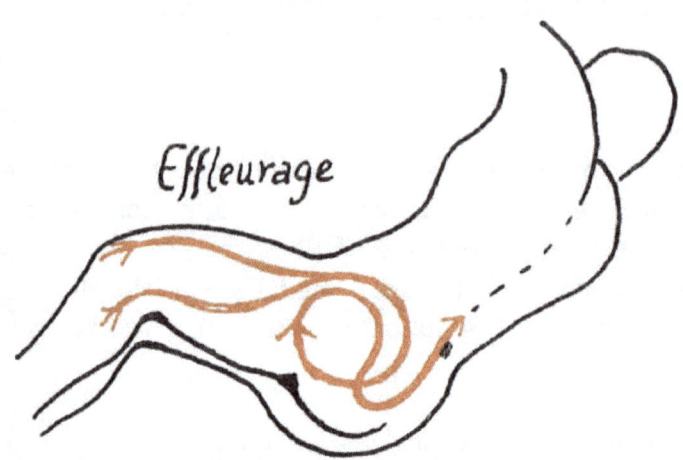

Effleurage

1. Effleurage. The masseur stands by the side of the hip. He collects with both hands the streams from the thigh, circulates on the buttock and leads the stroke a short distance up the back, solidly and without swinging off.

2. Kneading. First the back muscles of the thigh kneading toward oneself with special kneading of the region of the tuberosity of ischium with the ball of the thumb and fingers. This is followed by the treatment of the lateral and front parts of the quadriceps with continuation in circular movements around the trochanter and around the buttocks.

3. Airy Kneading ("Walken") of the thigh and, as in the case of the leg from behind, warming circles from the thigh up to the buttocks. Here, too, a short treatment of the lower back may be added. Ending stroke quite short as at the start.

Massage of the Back

Duration 10 to 15 minutes. Position: lying comfortably on the stomach, shoulders lying on the table as flat as possible, small support for the forehead or hands under the forehead for easy breathing. In the case of hollow lower back put a cushion under the abdomen, don't forget the foot roll.

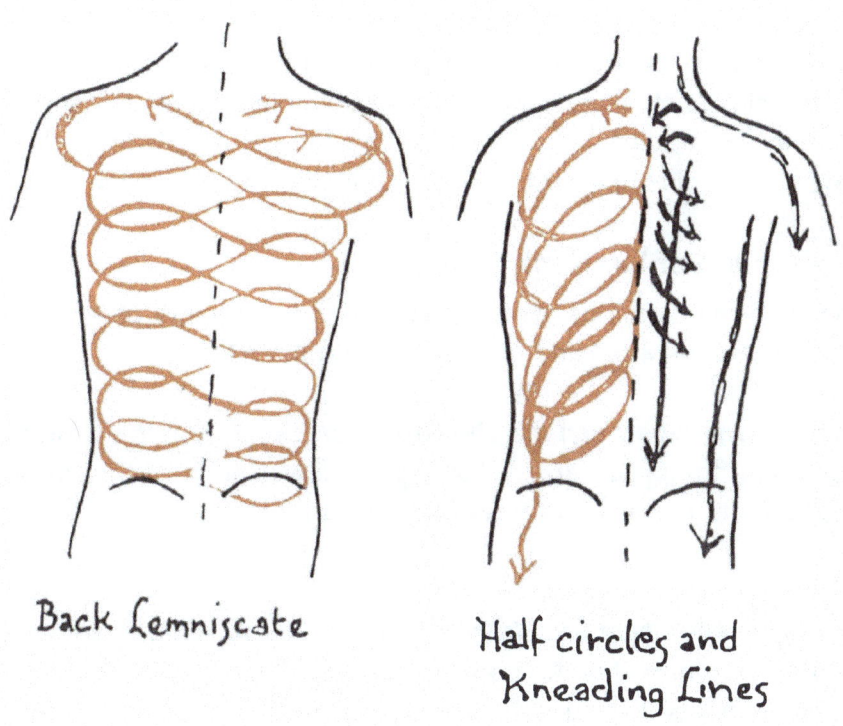

Back Lemniscate

Half circles and Kneading Lines

1. Effleurage. Large warming lemniscate movement with both hands several times downward and upward, passing over into some long down strokes right and left of the spinal column.

2. Loosening of the neck through small circular frictions on the muscles at the back of the head between the mastoid processes and along the occipital bone where the nerve foramina lie. Finish with loosening grip passing over into careful stretching of the neck muscles, vertebra after vertebra (so-called rabbit grip).

3. Loosening treatment of each side of the neck by itself with delicate kneading on the side of the neck downward over the shoulder into the upper arm.

4. Treatment of the region of the seventh cervical vertebra, loosening circular movement, from there descending loosening kneading, first with shifting of the phases, then without the latter on both sides of the spinal column (so-called fir tree) with following firm down strokes. All movements are round, parts of a circle.

5. Kneading along the whole back in four lines, the flanks and right and left of the spine.

6. Warmth circles over half the back without stroking of the spaces between the ribs, emphasized conclusion through light kneading of the hip. Here also a treatment of the lower back may be added. This is ended by long down strokes with downward emphasis over the whole back, strengthening uprightness.

Diversion Massage of the Neck

Duration: 10 to 15 minutes. Position: The patient sits at a table or with a pillow on his lap, supporting the lower arms and thereby relaxing the neck.

1. Loosening the region between the shoulder blades and from the middle of the spine toward outside into the upper arm, following the lower edge of the trapezius. Do not push the movements upward into the head, but always work toward the outside and downward.

2. Muscular origins and nerve exits from ear to ear. The masseur stands sideways and lightly supports the forehead of the patient with the left hand. With the right hand, as in back massage, he treats the muscular origins and places of nerve exit from ear to ear. In addition, pulling away the neck muscles vertebra after vertebra.

3. Loosening of the sides of the neck and kneading over the shoulder height down into the deltoid muscle. Out strokes in front of the ear, past the side veins of the neck and over the shoulder into the upper arm.

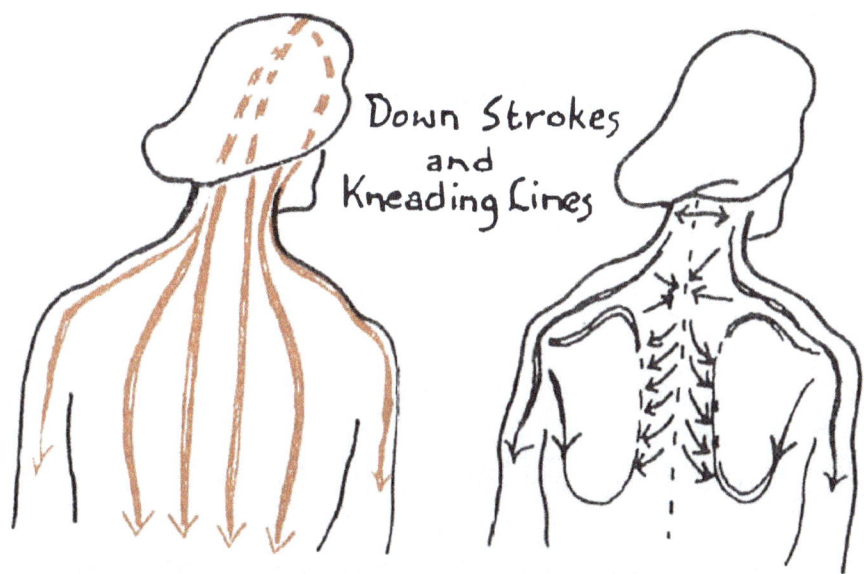

4. Treatment of the region of the seventh cervical vertebra, followed by descending, loosening kneading right and left of the spine (the so-called *fir tree*, as in the back massage).

5. The masseur again stands at the side, one hand supports the shoulder from the front, the other kneads *in circles around the entire shoulder blade*, first lightly, then fuller and deeper.

6. Finally there follow concluding down strokes upon three lines (see drawing above). These down strokes have to be made especially quietly, firmly, and carefully.

In this whole treatment care has to be taken that the patient must be able to sit completely quietly, he must not be shaken or pushed, since this treatment is chiefly used in a tendency to migraine and other congestions in the head.

Knee Massage

Duration about 20 minutes. A knee treatment must always be preceded by a light treatment of the thigh. Position: Leg on knee roll. Always treat both knees.

1. Effleurage. Above the knee, sideways, and at the underside lightly lifting. Flat ascending circular movements from the upper third of the calf, with special consideration of the hollow of the knee up to the underside of the thigh. Then lay the knee upon a roll.

2. Light kneading of the quadriceps above the knee, and of the muscles right and left past the patella.

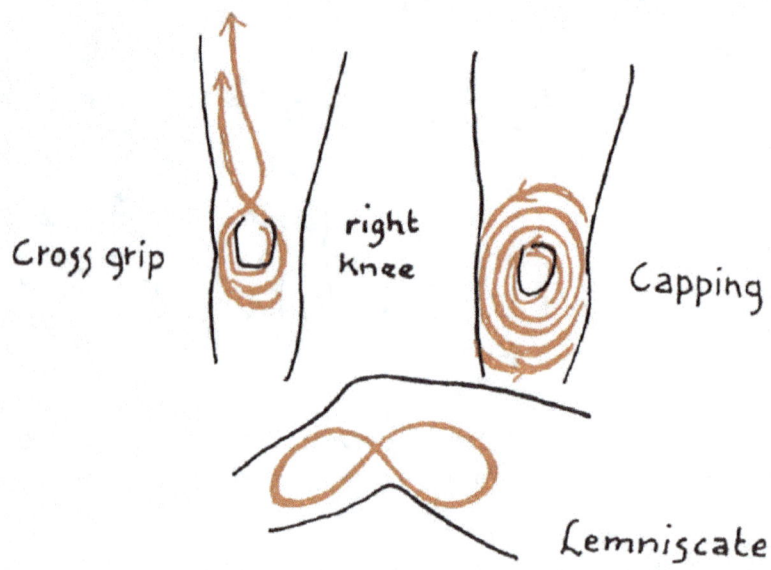

3. Careful frictions around the patella in two semicircles, while the second hand supports the patella. This is followed by the outstroke combining the frictions, beginning with crossed thumbs below the patella, then past it sideways, crossing above again and passing along the quadriceps.

4. Warming circular movements over the knee toward outside (formation of the warmth cap as on the shoulder), taking care not to displace the patella.

Foot Massage

Duration: 20 minutes for both feet. Position: Sitting or lying. Foot treatment must be preceded by a light treatment of the calf. Take the foot firmly in both hands, both thumbs lying on the inside.

1. Airy Kneading ("Walken") to warm and loosen the whole foot, beginning with the toes as far upward as possible. Several times forward and backward.

2. Stirrup grip for the treatment of the back of the foot with both thumbs. The spaces between the toes are treated one after the other with friction up to the middle of the foot.

3. Kneading of the outer edge of the foot. One hand remains lying on the back of the foot, warming it.

4. Turning to the treatment of the arch, taking hold firmly, and treating the entire arch of the foot with thumb and ball of the thumb from the ball of the foot to the heel.

5. Friction of the heel, loosening and warming.

6. Ascending circular frictions right and left of the Achilles tendon, descending in front over the malleolus. Smooth round stroke follows. Repeat this several times.

These six grips are carried out repeatedly forward and backward. Conclusion as in the first grip. Further special treatments of the toes do not belong to the basic form.

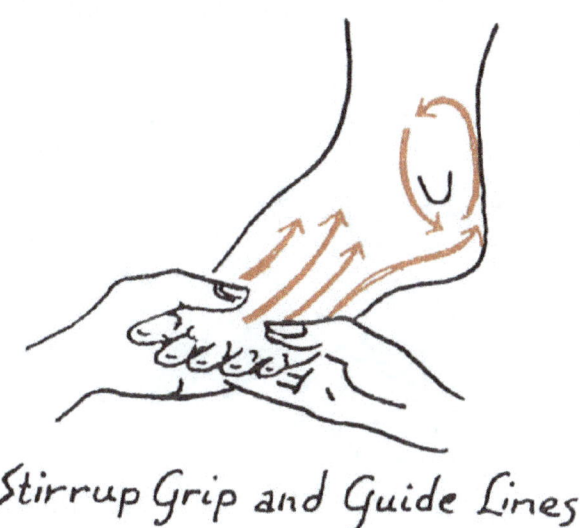

Stirrup Grip and Guide Lines

Hand Massage

The massage of the hand is carried out like that of the foot. Numbers 5 and 6 are eliminated. Instead the treatment of the back of the hand is continued to the wrist, adding in most cases a special treatment of the fingers.

Massage of the Abdomen

Duration: 15 to 20 minutes. Position: Lying comfortably on the back with knee support.

1. *Thorough stroking out of the colon* in two phases, first transverse colon and descending branch, then from the caecum upward with the edge of the little finger.

2. *Both colonic flexures*. This stroking is followed by the treatment of left and right colonic flexures with circular frictions, first flat, then carefully going deeper. All movements are carried out slowly and softly, tensions are slowly loosened.

3. *Around the navel*. Stimulation of the small intestine through spiral-like circles around the navel, followed by a soft kneading.

4. *Kneading of the abdominal musculature downward* from somewhat above the ribs to the symphysis in four lines.

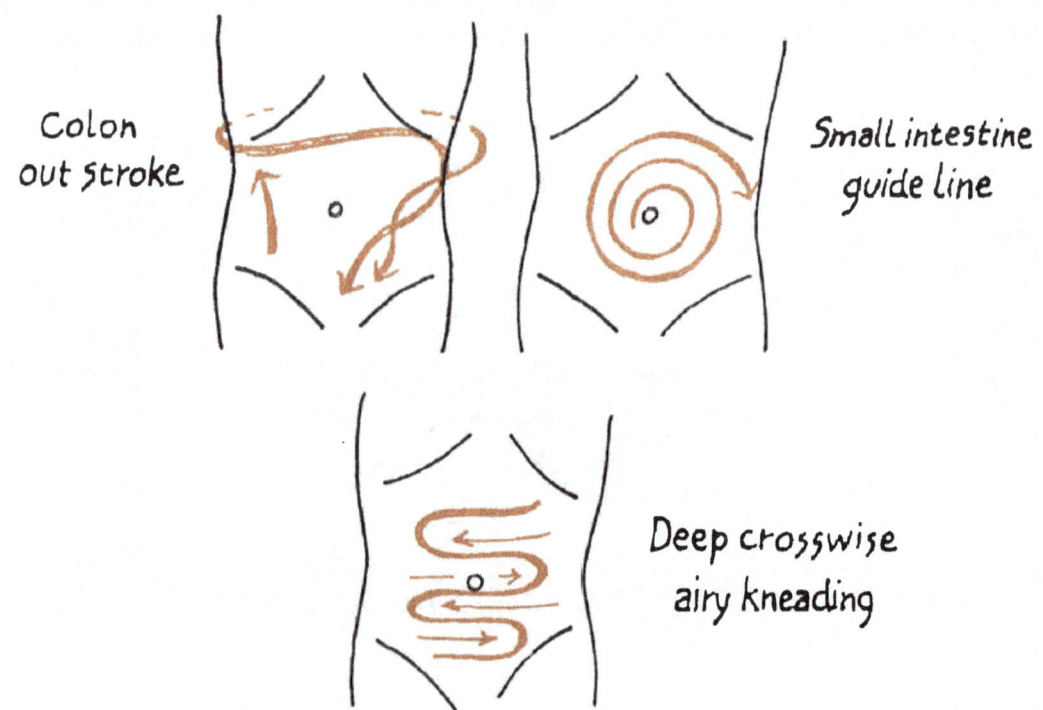

5. Deep airy kneading ("Walken") movements across the whole abdomen (see diagram on previous page).

6. Circular frictions pulling forward from the quadratus lumborum and ending in the colon out stroke. A comprehensive out stroke ends the abdominal massage.

Head Massage

Position: Sitting, Introduction: A short *diversion massage of the neck* without the movements around the shoulder blade. Minimal use of oil.

After the introduction cover the neck and start at the muscle origins at the *back of the head. Frictions from ear to ear* and a small distance up to back of the head. A few soft, broad neck grips at the end.

This is followed by small frictions around the ear, up in front over the origin of the facial nerve and down in the back over the mastoid process. The *external ear* is lightly pulled away from the head and thoroughly kneaded with two fingers.

Loosening of the *entire scalp* through flat movements with the palms of the hand. (Each hand on one half of the head. After the friction with the finger tips, repeat the flat grip.

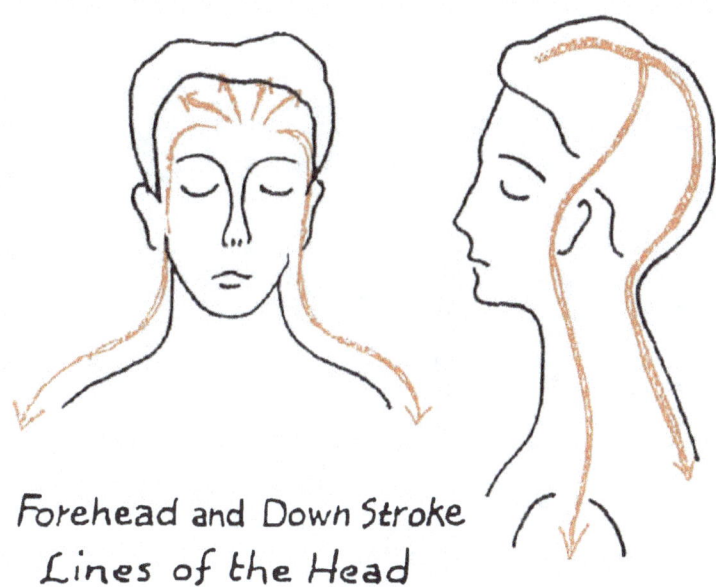

Forehead and Down Stroke Lines of the Head

The *forehead* is treated with ray-like frictions starting upward from the root of the nose. *Eyebrow stroke* in front of the ear downward. The same under the eye outward over the zygoma. The out stroke: pull up from the back of the nose over the zygoma (slit eye) and likewise in front of the ear downward.

Very light, loose frictions over the closed eye from the inner corner, outward may be introduced, also frictions from the point of the chin to the angle of the jaw.

Returning to the forehead with broad, flat frictions, which continue in the flat grips for the loosening of the scalp. Down strokes: from the hair line *past the ear in front* into the upper arm and from the forehead backward into the back, lightly on the hair, firm in the back.

PART THREE

THE APPLICATION OF RHYTHMICAL MASSAGE

21.

EMBROCATION OF THE ORGANS

With this chapter we begin to make suggestions for the treatment of certain groups of diseases. It is self-evident that every physician or masseur will have to revise or change these indications according to the individual state of his patient. These indications, therefore, do not have the character of a prescription, they point only to the situation of the members of being in general and to the possibilities of handling the specific case. The Science of the Spirit and here, in a narrower sense, the spiritual-scientific knowledge of man, describes the interrelationships investigated by Rudolf Steiner. This science in no way claims absolute authority, but its results cannot be properly used by those who do not understand them. Someone with an open mind who occupies himself with it in an unprejudiced way for a longer period of time, will find that it grows within him into a spiritually logical coherent picture of world and man that enables him to act out of knowledge in his own professional field.

Within Rhythmical Massage the *organ rubbings* take a special position. The masseur should not carry them out without agreement with the doctor, if they are not prescribed.

They were introduced by Rudolf Steiner as 'gentle massage of the spleen,' (Sixteen Lectures to Doctors, Dornach, 1921). *Gentle massage of the spleen* acts in an equalizing way upon the *breaking down processes of the nerve-sense life* and at the same time improves the *activity of instincts*. These permit something of the wisdom of the lower astral body which inwardly serves the metabolism to press up into consciousness. It is a gentle waking up of the organic function of the spleen which unites everything we take up into us with our individual rhythm. Foreign rhythms inherent in the food substances through their own nature must by no means be taken over. The spleen 'knows' what is good for us and what is not beneficial.

All the other organs have their differentiated task and unique function that can be awakened through gentle massage of the region under which the organ lies. Originally these massages were carried out only by the physicians during their visits. Later on it was found to be desirable also to train the nurses in these procedures; indeed, even to add an organ rubbing into the massage treatment.

Rudolf Steiner states in regard to the spleen that one must not go too far with this massage in order not to obtain the opposite result; this holds good for all the other organs. Besides the spleen, liver, kidney and heart are treated. Naturally, warm circular movements with a concluding character toward inside could be carried out. This is done with little children where the space is so small. With adults an increase can be obtained through the more breathing motion of the lemniscate. The large organs are special places for the ego activity, they have always to be within a warmth sheath in order to function properly. Therefore in an organ treatment the second, that is, the left hand always lies lightly on or below the patient as if one were to insert the organ into the warmth stream from hand to hand. For the same reason it is advisable to carry out the movement of the lemniscate belonging to the sun. The liver forms a certain exception. Here two organs, liver and gall process, are interwoven. The breathing character will best be reached here through expanding and contracting circles or spirals. The lemniscate cannot be used here because of the shape of the ribs. In organ rubbings the hand has to make especially good contact and while completely relaxed follow the plastic surface of the body and work rhythmically like the beating of a bell. To imagine the sound element helps to gain the insight that also the organ has to sound in the depths.. One should try to gain the *resonance to the outer movement*. The duration of a rubbing is one to two minutes. One should, however, not massage by following a clock. Gradually the masseur acquires a sure feeling as to when the organ is 'satisfied,' as it were, and when the treatment has to end with a conscious out stroke.

Since the *metals* are those substances in the earth through which cosmic forces work out of *the planetary world*, having originated through the radiating activity of the planets into the earth in the past, it becomes clear that *metal ointments* are used for the rubbing of organs. The choice of ointments must be made by the physician since it is not a question of fixed mechanical arrangement. Naturally, other ointments may be used which bring the process into a special direction; that is to say, which affect one of the members of man's being in a particular way.

The Spleen Rubbing

Since the spleen lies behind the stomach and on the side, the rubbing consists of a lemniscate with large upper loop on the lower rib cage toward the back. The lower loop of the lemniscate lies on the flank and is much smaller; indeed, it may be contracted into a breathing turning point. The second hand lies on the right side of the upper abdomen, diagonally. The organ rubbing, simple as it may look, demands the full attention of the masseur in order to prevent a mechanical motion. It must musically vary in tempo and be very warm.

Today almost all patients need a spleen massage since in the rush and hurry of our city life nobody, as Rudolf Steiner stated, possesses a normal function of the spleen. It goes without saying, however, that it is especially needed in all *metabolic weaknesses, nutritional disturbances* and wherever the *predominating breaking down processes* of the nerve sense system have led to light or serious intoxications. (See Chapter "The Hand"). This is the case in most chronic diseases which are accompanied by spasms, congestions, sclerotic tendencies, depository and degenerative phenomena, right up to deformations.

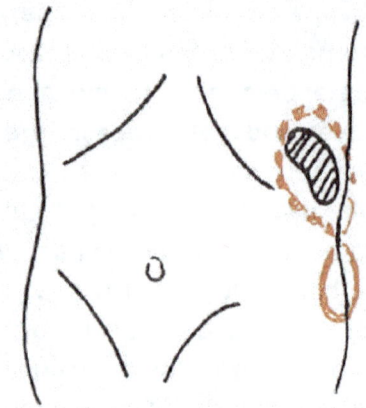

The upper loop lies posteriorly

In most cases one will not only rub the spleen, but one will add the liver treatment.

The Liver Rubbing

Position: Lying on the back as in the rubbing of the spleen. It consists of expanding and contracting circles, the centre of which lies in the region of the gallbladder. The second hand lies on the back side of the liver (see drawing on next page).

The liver rubbing, too, has a very broad field of indication. The liver is the great alchemist of our metabolism. Normally it has a raised temperature, thus a very active warmth organism, which prepares the way for the ego into the complicated metabolism in order to keep it on the height necessary for the human organism. Any decrease in this regard would mean the sinking down to the level of the animal or even vegetative region. The liver forms the *center of the warmth processes* in metabolism which we need for the unfolding of our will in movement. It controls the *metabolism of the musculature* by mobilizing the sustances necessary for the unfolding of movement.

On the other hand, it synthesizes the substances producing urine and is active in *detoxification* of the metabolism. It prepares the gall which, on its part, must be admixed very early to the nutritional stream so that the ego organization can accompany the transformation of substances from the very beginning; for the gall is reabsorbed in the intestine, thus passing through its own circulation. Since the liver with the portal vein receives all the blood from the intestinal region, it is the organ predominantly active in the upbuilding processes. The liver, too, like the spleen, is exposed to much damage through our culture. The chemical treatment of soil and food stuffs, alcoholism and nicotine are components burdening the metabolism, let alone the psychic burdens which many people 'swallow,' as it were. Since the liver is the

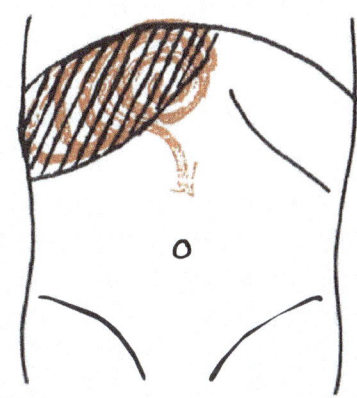

Spiral Winding Out and In

chief support of our will activity we see today more often than in times past a decisive paralysis of the will, of the individual capacity of resolution and force of action. Liver and gall processes lead spirit and soul deeply into metabolism, into the fluid man. If they do not master the transformation of substances, congestions with depressions and a bilious mood arise. There are many stages leading to deeper disturbances and finally to complete paralysis of will. This is the case with the so-called 'mentally ill.' However, it is never the mind, the spirit, that is ill, but the body fetters the spirit and prevents it from manifesting itself normally. Our consciousness is a mirroring process in the body. If the body is deformed, the mirror distorted, as it were, psychic anomalies appear, the causes of which are to be found in the body, in the most delicate metabolic disturbances.

A slight liver congestion lies at the basis of almost every 'emotional upset.' Disputatiousness, obstinacy and cramping up of the will are frequently simultaneous phenomena. The discharge in the choleric fit is but the swinging of the pendulum toward the other side which concerns the gall process to a greater degree.

The rubbing of the liver will be of beneficial result in *indigestion, in liver congestions*, in the so-called *vegetative dystonia, in constipation and flatulence*. Furthermore, it will *stimulate the warmth organism* in all kinds of *circulatory disturbances* starting with chronically cold hands and feet right up to *serious arteriosclerosis with tendency toward gangrene*.

Liver rubbing is to be recommended in metabolic disturbances such as *rheumatism, arthritis, damage to the lumbar vertebra, diabetes*, etc.

Liver rubbings have been successful in *headaches* connected with sluggishness of the intestines, frequently found with school children at the age of four to fourteen where normally astral body and ego ought to descend deeper into the metabolic process but are prevented from doing so (for instance, through overburdening in school).

A special field for the application of liver and spleen rubbings are all disturbances in the thoracic cavity in the sense of the handicapped breathing, such as *asthma, emphysema, chronic bronchitis* and so on, also *anginous heart trouble*. Here the treatment of the upper abdomen as such is always of unburdening effect.

Finally, we should like to mention that we can conceive of liver rubbing as an *aid to incarnation with weak, anaemic children, bed wetters*, and also in *recovery* after *infectious diseases*. Liver rubbing has a special significance in psychiatry. The rubbing, carried out warmly and rhythmically, can bring about a *collecting and embodying of the loosened members of man's being*, also a lifting out of depression of the submerged members of man's being to a medium, rhythmical, healthy interplay in metabolism. Rhythmical Massage has the advantage of acting beneficially toward both sides, the side of too much binding and also a too loose cohesion of the members of man's being, thereby leading the functions to a healthy harmony.

The Kidney Rubbing

The kidney rubbing is a double lemniscate carried out with both hands in counter-movement in such a way that without too much pressure the region above the kidneys is thoroughly warmed. The out stroke at the end is generally downward, it can, however, be upward if the kidney radiation is to be specially stimulated. The out strokes are to be done quietly and briefly.

The kidney has, in the interplay of the great organs that signify our inner world system, a task in the upbuilding metabolism as well as the task of eliminating the surplus of breaking down substances that results in the balancing of breaking down and upbuilding processes; that is to say, it has to be active in the breaking down metabolism.

Naturally, this is expressed summarily. The kidney helps in this regard the harmonizing heart function. The secretion of urine is not its only task. It has higher tasks which are connected with respiration and the air organism. Since it uses most oxygen it creates the hunger for air. In the lower man it is the *organ of radiation for the astral body* which acts via the air organism into the fluid and solid element, and in this way permeates us with the capacity of sensation, in other words, it ensouls the organs. This *kidney radiation* is supersensible, described by Rudolf Steiner as an inner light formation in which the astral body works. This explains the close connection of the kidney to consciousness and the life of feeling. Kidney diseases know both sides of deviation from soul equilibrium: the *irritable emotional*, the unrest, but also the *stupor* and unconsciousness in complete failure. The kidney is a highly sensitive organ and extremely sensitive to cold. The great organ systems can properly be grasped only in their total interplay since the totality always takes part in their physiological processes.

Thus in the upbuilding process of human protein, for example, the total inner world system participates, as it is described in Dr. Rudolf Hauschka's book *Nutrition*, in the chapter "Formation of Protein by the Organs."

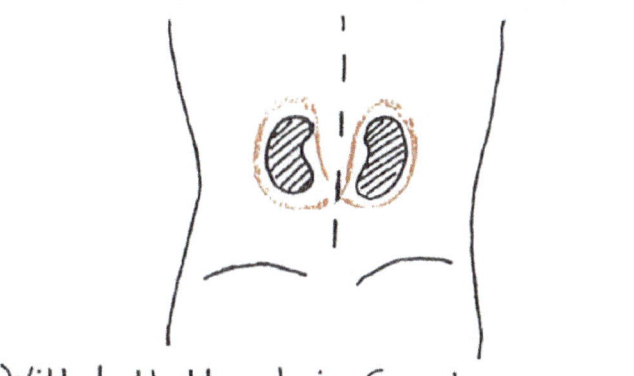

With both Hands in Countermovement

Kidney rubbing has proved itself especially beneficial in the case of *weak kidney activity with excretory deficiency*, in the *tendency toward stone formation*, in *sinking of the kidney*, in *kidney congestion*, accompanied by *eczemas or allergic rashes*, also irritation of the eyes; also, in chronic lumbago and *rheumatic phenomena*.

In every treatment by massage, attention has to be paid to sufficient kidney function. Through massage many deposits re-enter the blood stream, and if there is not enough excretion through the kidney, the result is a dulled consciousness right up to migraine headache. In these cases the pauses between the treatments must be longer and the massage has to be very gentle. It is always advisable for the masseur to take this into account. Every *inflammatory kidney affliction* is naturally a definite *contra-indication*. The frequency and length of kidney rubbings is to be chosen carefully, better too short than too long. Attention has to be paid especially to warmth formation, and not too much ointment or oil should be used in order to prevent loss of contact.

The Heart Rubbing

We have learned to know the heart as the center, the sun of the inner world system. Through shifting of the balance it may experience disturbances from two sides; first, through the encroaching of the formative, mineralizing forces of the upper man, and, second, through the reaching up of the loosening forces of metabolism. There are, therefore, two kinds of heart rubbing. At the basis of both treatments there lies, logically, the lemniscate as the form of movement especially ascribed to the sun.

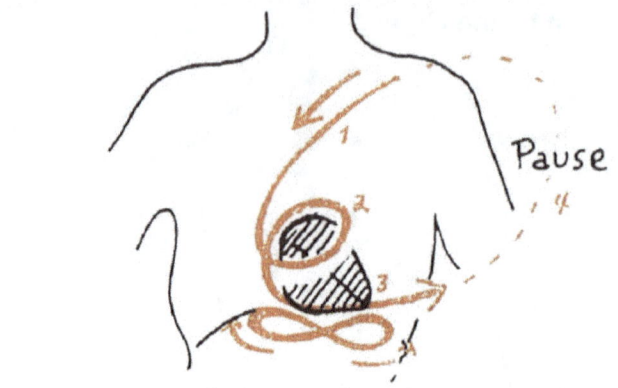

Calming and Stimulating Heart Rubbing

First the lemniscate is led from above downward into a calming effect, it is a turned-in lemniscate that expresses the calming inwardness of forces but it is also determined through the shape of the body. Rhythm is essential here; it is a rhythm of four phases; three phases lie on the body, the fourth is the pause.

The stimulating heart rubbing is a horizontal lemniscate below the chest in the two-phase rhythm of a bell. It is precisely in the heart rubbing that these forms must not be applied like an abstract formation; on the contrary, they must be fitted to the form of the breast, producing a soft, harmonious, rhythmical movement with good and warm contact, but not with pressure.

This second, stimulating heart rubbing, is a somewhat faster, more concentrated movement in contrast to the calming stroke of the upper loop in the first rubbing which descends from the height of the shoulder.

The ego is anchored in the blood, in the middle man; however, it is supported mainly by the heart. Thus the heart in its higher parts has special centrally-human tasks. Here the ego feeling arises. It relies upon a special center in the etheric body that is present in the heart sphere. Heart experience is always representative for the whole. Our *feeling of self* mirrors the state of the heart, it vanishes if the heart breaks down and may lead to the *feeling of absolute annihilation*, which appears in attacks of *angina pectoris*. The heart is the place where physical warmth as the highest level of all physiological processes can pass over into soul warmth. Thus the heart is our *organ of spiritualization*. It is described by Rudolf Steiner as the sphere in man where the physical can be etherized; that is, spiritualized, but also where the spiritual can manifest physically. On this quality rests the formation of conscience, which signifies the mirroring in the heart of a moral judgment pronounced by a spiritual power higher than our ordinary ego. The feeling of responsibility also belongs in this context. We might also say that the heart harbors a force of *transfiguration*, a force to idealize and warm up to ideals. Even noble anger, that flames up in the face of injustice, relies on the heart organism and not so much on liver and gall, for it is not bitter, but like a purifying flame. The ether center of the heart is the source of all creative forces. In the heart there rests the future of man. If that were not so, would it be permissible to call the heart an inner sun? The dead knowing of such cosmic relationships has no meaning if it does not lead to an entirely new science of man that kindles knowledge which opens entirely new perspectives and which transform the knower.

Rudolf Steiner once described the sun as the *flaming guarantor of our liberty*, but also the place where our *misused freedom* is conglomerated into our *destiny* from life to life. "The sun is the flame in which freedom appears phosphorically in the universe and it is, at the same time, the substance in which, as though in conglomerated ashes, misused freedom bakes itself together as destiny in order to be able to be effective until this destiny itself can pass over into the flame of liberty."* The ego that relies on the heart can liberate itself from the compulsion of the urges of the material body and also from the compulsion of reason in Schiller's sense; that is to say, from the urge of substance and the urge of form, and it is able to perform free deeds of love out of the center; it can, in spite of all expectation of the intellect, pardon and give, it can through this alone permeate destiny with sun forces, permeate it with the Christ.

This book is written for people who through their professional studies have learned the anatomical- physiological facts in the sense of modern science. This science, however, eliminates the higher man, and the extended view must be directed upon the man of spirit and soul, but not solely upon it, but also upon its dependence upon the body. *The way spirit connects itself with matter and reveals itself through it, is the subject of the western science of the spirit.* It fully acknowledges the results of natural-scientific observation but it must add the results of spiritual observation. The higher man was always known in all ancient cultures, in eastern and western schools of wisdom; it is, however, the task of Middle Europe to develop the ideas regarding the way in which body and soul are connected and where the bridges are to be looked for. This task has been fulfilled by Rudolf Steiner.

Let us return to heart massage. The indications are easily to be read from what has been presented. An excitable heart may be calmed, a slack one stimulated. Again it is a question of leading to a middle rhythmical activity. In more serious disturbances the treatment of the heart will not suffice; in *anginal disturbances* one has to make *diverting grips* at the periphery, in heart rate accelerations leading to the frequently occurring

---

*   Rudolf Steiner, *The Spiritual Individualities of the Planets*, 'The Golden Blade,' Rudolf Steiner Press, London, 1966.

paroxysmal tachycardia one has to carry out *formative grips* on the lower extremities which aid incarnation.

The treatment of the heart may never be separated from a treatment of the entire circulation and must always be included in it.

22.

THE SPINAL COLUMN AND ITS TREATMENT

The diseases of the spinal column are a phenomenon that has strongly increased in recent decades and occupies an ever larger space in the practice of massage. As long as one considers the damages of the spine as a mechanical problem according to our technologically inclined thinking, we shall not do justice to this organ serving human uprightness. It is necessary to consider the *spinal column as a functional unit*, in the upbuilding and maintaining of which the whole human being participates.

In order to understand the special way of treating the spine in massage with its emphasis on the principle of the lemniscate, we shall make some preliminary remarks about the anatomy and evolutionary history of this organ.

The archetype of the entire skeleton, the vertebra-rib system, from which the whole skeleton can be derived through metamorphoses, is to be understood as a lemniscatic formation holding the balance between cosmic weightlessness and earthly gravity.

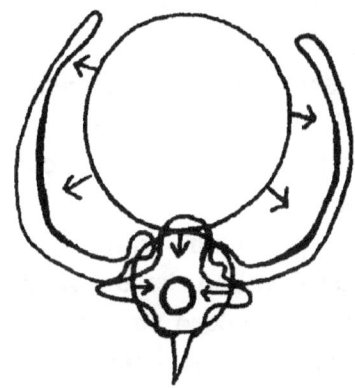

The hovering rib and the contracted vertebra form together a lemniscatic archetype which varies as we move up and down the spine. In the middle, vertebra and rib are harmoniously shaped. Upward, the light rib principle increasingly predominates in the vertebrae until finally in the atlas, the cervical vertebra, only the hovering ring remains; downward, the bodies and the contracting principle become ever mightier until finally only the coccyx with its salt-cubelike form remains.

The spinal column is the formation holding together all the otherwise separated parts of the skeleton. Just as the physical body forms the vessel for the three higher principles of life, soul, and spirit, so the spinal column holds together these three principles in a likeness. Moreover, these principles play a special part in the upbuilding of the spine. The spine contains an *etheric principle of growth* like a plant which grows from node to node. Its leaves unfold in the ribs and finally it produces the head like a blossom. Out of this the *astral principle* shapes a *hollow form*, provides the orientation in space, and joins the spinal column powerfully to the inner world system with its strong blood supply. *The principle of polarity* in every direction, also *the mobility*, are expressions of the astral-animal stage of the structure. The whole, however, is subject to the *ego-organization*. This lifts the structure up into the human, stamps upon the spinal column the universal, cosmic measures, creates the *functional unity* and takes hold of the organ with the power of uprightness and bestows on it the functional form of the double S-curve. It goes without saying that from the very start these principles are active and interlock in the inception of the vertebra.

The life body permeated by rhythm is always the mediator between the formative principles of soul and spirit and the physical. The creative principle, in this case the ego, always uses rhythmical processes if matter is to be formed. The spine is an example of interpenetrating formative rhythms, the details of which are shown in Karl König's articles mentioned in the chapter, "Metamorphoses of the Skeleton."

I should still like to draw attention to a special fact in the formation of the vertebrae, as illustrated in the drawing on the following page.

At the twenty-first day of the development of the embryo there arise within a few days alongside the Chorda dorsalis the *forty-four cellular collections of the archetypal vertebra* arranged in pairs. They consist of the *sclerotome*, the inception of the skeleton, and the *myotome*, the inception of the muscular system. The entire structure originates in the middle germ layer.

The sclerotomes have a fine split in the middle. The eventual vertebrum arises now through a shifting. In the splits young tissue remains. From it there arise the *intervertebral discs* with their jelly-like core enclosed in a ring-like fibrocartilage and having the *form of a biscuit*. This form is a forerunner of the lemniscate within the series of the Cassini curves belonging to it. The relationship of the archetypal vertebra to the final vertebra could be expressed musically as a *series of seconds*, the intersounding of two sound forms, in our case the being shifted into one another of two formative rhythms.

Artistic conceptions rather than purely abstract considerations can be an aid for the understanding of organic formations. In this case we have to take into account Rudolf Steiner's characterization of *music* as an *ego power that has moved down half a stage into the realm of the astral, the soul*. Thereby music arises just as *painting*, the colorfully pictorial, arises through the soul power dipping down half a stage into *the etheric*, and *sculpture* arises through the *laws of life*, the etheric plane, descending half a stage into *the physical*.

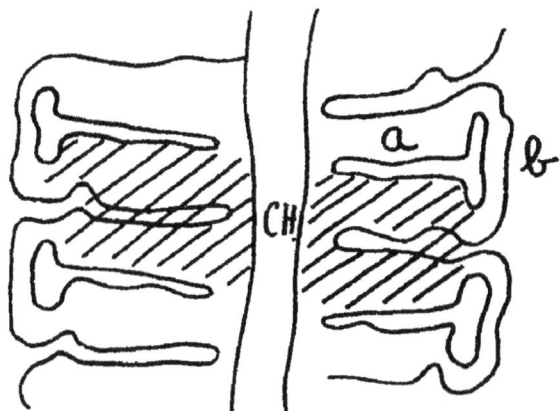

Hatched Lines = Position of the Later Vertebrae

If with such thoughts we look upon this shifting of formation in the spine, 'the latter characterizes itself as an organ quite especially subjected to the musical ego force. This becomes evident at once, for otherwise the tendency to erectness, a function of the ego, could not take hold of the spinal column. It is interesting to note in this connection that even animals in hearing music that contains this ego power try to achieve erectness.

Moreover, Rudolf Steiner describes how the breathing life transplants itself into the cerebro-spinal fluid and produces within it soft rising and falling movements which pass through the variously formed intervening space. Thereby the whole structure resembles a musical instrument. In the ancient mysteries this was called the 'lyre of Apollo.' The mysterious happenings around the nervous system swimming in the fluid in connection with breathing is the result of man's being permeated by soul and spirit. On the paths of music, that is to say, of the stellar order, the human body is raised upon the stage of the ego. When in the course of the ancient cultures in the Greek age the 'I' for the first time awakens in human consciousness, the leading inspirer is Apollo with the lyre. Today we do not even have an inkling of what a decisive role music and its quality plays for man. If we were not structured according to the laws of music that stem from the realm of the stars, our bodies could not receive an ego.

Let us mention the intervertebral disc. The disc is an arrested remains of the core of the archetypal vertebra in which are intermixed excrescent remains of the chorda dorsalis. Thus it is a still plastic, youthful tissue. In the chest part the discs are the lowest and of equal height. In the neck and lumbar region they are ventrally considerably higher which corresponds to lordosis. All intervertebral discs together equal more than one fourth of the entire length of the spine. At this point I should like to report on x-ray observations of the walking human being. We find that with every step all the vertebrae perform a lemniscate movement on the individual discs. This movement is smallest at the top of the spine. Only the head remains quiet. The physical imprint of this characteristic movement is the hollow formed by the lemniscate visible on every disc. The spinal processes move very gently to and fro. The general impression is that of the fin of a fish moving in the water from above downward. This report shows clearly to what small degree the movements of the living human being are mechanical but how they are rather controlled by the formative forces of the etheric body, weaving in the fluid element.

From all this we shall readily understand that the spinal column is affected if the formative impulses of spirit and soul partially withdraw from it. It has repeatedly been observed that the delicate shiftings in it may also become the cause for ailments far removed from it like *arthrosis* and *arthritis*, even disturbances of the inner organs such as *stomach*, *pancreas*, *heart*, and so on. Normally, the bone connection of the spine is held by taut ligaments which, naturally, fail in such cases.

Acute or chronic concussions to which we are constantly exposed through our culture, *are most damaging to the spine*. Here we must not think merely of mechanical concussions of which there are a great number through man's close connection with machines and through our concrete paths and our hard gait. But we must not forget modern *beat music* with its *counter rhythms* which, in the longer term, is able to shake the sheath for our instrument of spiritualization, for the lyre of Apollo. We can see already that not the individual thoughtful ego but foreign powers seize the soul and the body when human masses expose themselves to this 'music.' Furthermore, damaging influences occur through *wrong nutrition*, through *the effects of cold and over-exertion*, if there exists a hereditary weakness of the whole organism. Last but not least, there stands behind everything a soul attitude that through *negation of the spiritual individuality* and through *paralyzing of individual initiative* in a culture of comfort, insurance policies and authoritative egalitarianism does not permit the ego of man to be active in the right way. Very often social warmth, which permits the one ego to awaken through the other, thereby warming and unfolding itself, is lacking. In short, there are reasons enough why in our time the most central part of our skeleton runs the risk of decaying and increasingly needs medical treatment.

While in the field of remedies a basic therapy has been made possible through the Wala *intervertebral disc preparations* containing bamboo, in Rhythmical Massage it is possible to gain extensive improvement of the function and a strengthening of the improvement once it is gained.

Every case must be treated individually. Principally, after an introductory orienting massage of the back that may be light and loosening, softly avoiding the painful spots, a repeated purely *lemniscatic treatment* with ever decreasing forms is indicated over the whole back downwards. If in back massage the complaint is located in the cervical or lumbar region, the emphasis of the treatment has to be put accordingly above or below. In any case, also in cervical disturbances the root of the spine must be treated through careful, warming massage of the hips and the lower back. *Abdominal massage* with the *abdominal upstroke* and concluding *rubbing of the liver* may be added; they bring about a better blood supply through the metabolism. A really lasting improvement can only be reached if *streaming arm and leg massages* are added in order to bring to the organ spine forces from above and below and again to insert it properly into the general circulation of life.

The practice of avoiding the painful spots has been from the beginning and remains a main principle. Only after improvement has taken place may the ill regions be treated more intensively. In the case of a decided *damage to the cervical vertebra* the *neck massage* with its relieving pull-away grips of the ligamentum nuchae is of special importance. The grips must be carried out slowly for two to three minutes, vertebra after vertebra. Only when the neck and upper back have become loosened can forces be derived from arm massage. The leading off through neck massage is fortified by a few grips of the calves. Sometimes it is good to extend the treatment of the muscles at the back of the head to the region around the ears and upward to the scalp. Good outstrokes have to follow. Beside the liver rubbing, the *kidney rubbing* has proved beneficial in *damage of the cervical vertebra*. In the case of the lumbar syndrome, the massage of the hip and the streaming upward massage of the legs is of importance in order to lift the spinal column into the lightness of the living formative forces.

In the treatment of *weaknesses in posture* and *deformations*, also of *sclerosis* and similar ailments, the massage grips are placed as if one were dealing with a healthy spine. The down strokes especially do not follow the pathological form but play over it, impressing on the region of the spinal column a healthy form model. Terminal states of stiffening of the spine as in *ankylosing spondylitis* are treated under the following viewpoints: Warming and loosening massages of back, shoulders, and hips, supplying forces from arms and legs, lemniscatic collecting of the streams from above and below on the back which has been treated regularly with the loosening, soft grips of back massage. Introducing of abdominal massage as well as liver and kidney rubbings may be helpful.

Something that cannot be described and yet is an essential factor in the curative effect is the dosage. The customary treatment of massage lasting one half or even a whole hour does not apply in Rhythmical Massage. At the beginning very short treatments may be needed, which, however, may have discernible effects.

Intimate observation and experience are needed in order really to exhaust the possibilities of Rhythmical Massage.

23.

INDICATIONS FOR THE TREATMENT OF SPECIFIC CONDITIONS

1. General Effects of Rhythmical Massage

Because of its general effect of stimulating the life functions in all their stages, Rhythmical Massage will act beneficially in *convalescence*, in anemic and weakly constitutions, undernourishment and other *nutritional difficulties* and *developmental difficulties* of otherwise healthy young people and adults. To this we must add undefined ill feelings caused by damages incurred through modern civilization.

Since the health giving middle system is strengthened, the life body as mediator between spirit-soul and the body is awakened in its function, and the interplay of forces is made more fluid, healing can be brought about in many directions. Our cultural life leads to a certain stiffness and immobility of the etheric body caused by the use of chemical substances in our food and through radio, cinema, and television in our sense organs, mentioning only the most important aspects. Gradually the physical body is no longer fully permeated by soul and spirit. Rhythmical Massage brings about a better control of the physical body by the individuality. The patients feel themselves 'more erect' and freed of all kinds of dullness, making them more capable of dealing with the demands of life as the often subconscious feelings of inadequacy and faintness slowly vanish.

As is self-evident, among the general beneficial effects belong the *acceleration off the lymphatic stream* that prevents any congestion, and the *stimulation of the power of absorption* that prevents the falling away from life of parts of the fluid organism that form dead inclusions. Many people carry around a certain ballast of such lifeless parts of the water organism without paying attention to it and feel a great relief only after it has disappeared through treatment. The body as instrument of the soul is easier to handle so that its physical substance does not oppose the rhythms of the life body streaming through it with so many hindrances.

The fact that we constantly poison ourselves through our conscious life, that is, the life in the astral body and ego, making it necessary to equalize these conditions through detoxicating upbuilding and loosening processes originating in the ether body, leads to the necessary change of waking and sleeping.

This rhythm, too, normalizes itself frequently during a massage treatment which perhaps was started for quite different reasons. Since these slight poisoning states can call forth irritaion symptoms, manifesting psychically or bodily in itching of the skin and similar phenomena, a healthy calm ensues through the simple fact of the treatment with Rhythmical Massage. The simultaneous stimulation of the glandular activity brings about, among other things, a better appetite and better tolerance of food.

In such general treatments we do not give total massages but we alternate in the treatment of upper and lower man (arms, back and legs, abdomen or hips), the emphasis being varied according to the case. The treatment itself is rather short and moderately stimulating. All parts of the body are gradually permeated by rhythm and again connected with the life stream. Through gentle rubbings of spleen and liver (if it has been prescribed) the effect can be rounded off by thus gently stimulating the metabolism and aiding detoxification.

2. Bronchial Asthma

In bronchial asthma the following must be considered: The astral body giving the impulse to inbreathing does not descend sufficiently, causing congestion in the chest; exhalation becomes difficult. The *solidification tendency of the head invades the chest*, its form becomes rigid, the bronchial secretion becomes viscous; indeed, tendencies toward crystallization appear in it (Charcot-Leyden crystals). The terminal state of emphysema shows a barrel-like chest with diminished respiratory capacity.

Massage must draw the astral body into the metabolic limb region and thereby loosen the spasm in the chest space. We begin with the loosening of the *upper abdominal region* somewhat above and below the bow of the ribs. Since this region is often hard like a board, we begin with big, loosening grips which gradually become smaller and more intensive. There follow strong *calf grips*, and possibly *foot grips* which during an attack may bring relief. Then diverting *upper arm massages* and concentrating *back massages* are introduced, all grips must be warm, deep, and sucking. Later on there follows the treatment of the entire chest in front and in the back and the *exhalation strokes*, perhaps with vibration on both sides, from the upper back to the lower front, slightly compressing the lower part of the chest as an aid to exhalation, into this basic treatment massages of the calf and also of the whole leg are repeatedly inserted. Also the hip region including the lower back must be made pervious by deep kneading of the soft tissues. To this treatment belong also *abdominal massages* with special elaboration of deep airy transverse kneading and the cultivation of the M. Quadratus Lumborum. Liver and spleen rubbings accompany the entire treatment.

3. Angina Pectoris and Related Conditions

Begin exactly as in the treatment of asthma with loosening of the *upper abdomen*, perhaps of the whole abdomen with grips of the calf. Follow with arm massages downward with specially deep and sucking grips on the upper arm right down to the hand.

Later on, there follows a loosening of the entire chest wall (anterior and posterior). Calf and foot treatments are applied, alternating with upper arm and back massages including lower back and hips, aiding in deeper breathing.

Angina pectoris and related conditions are based on *disturbances of circulation of the heart* itself, from light to most serious cases. The coronary arteries are spastically contracted or are already degenerated and sclerotic, thereby endangering the nourishment of the heart muscle. Mostly lighter cases with anginal heart trouble are treated, but also more difficult cases may be treated successfully in the times between attacks. As in the case of asthma, the sclerosing forces of the head invade the rhythmical system, and all the stages of this shifting may be observed, from disturbances of rhythm and light spastic heart trouble up to serious coronary attacks with annihilating pain and fear of death. Therapy consists in diverting the astral body cramped up in the upper man downward, and loosening and making pervious the passages leading to the periphery and the limbs.

4. Disturbances in Arterial Blood Supply

Disturbance of arterial blood supply results from sclerosis of parts of the vascular system. In most cases the extremities, chiefly the legs, easily exposed to damage through cold, suffer from it. *Intermittent claudication*, *sensation of cold*, and attacks of *painful failure of the extremities* are the symptoms. These states of inadequate blood supply are serious for the reason that if they last too long the end of the limbs may mortify and the dreaded gangrene arises (Raynaud's disease).

These cases are in all stages, also the serious ones, much benefitted by the treatment with Rhythmical Massage. Because of the brittleness of the vessels all massages must be carried out carefully, with soft, sucking grips. One begins with the massage of back and *broad lower back treatment* in order to achieve a good warming of the root sphere of the limb. *The stimulation of the warmth organism* is the supreme goal. Right from the beginning, proceeding from the arms in the sense of the pentagram, one can stimulate the etheric streams in the leg. The leg itself will be treated directly only later, first it is gently kneaded. In the further course, the lower back, hip, and gradually the thigh are treated, again and again, producing warmth. In the more serious cases we remain at first with the treatment of the trunk. Only when the leg has become warm and capable of reaction can we gradually proceed from the thigh to the calf and possibly to the treatment of the foot.

From the very beginning the treatment includes deep, soft abdominal massages and, especially, liver rubbings.

The arm, if it is affected, is treated correspondingly. First, one has to make back and hip more permeable in order to bring about deeper breathing, then special attention is to be paid to the shoulder region and slowly one descends from upper to lower arm. A chill in the arm caused by driving a car with open windows and which is connected with paresthesia that leads to chronic epicondylitis, can be treated similarly with the addition of the lemniscatic treatment of the upper spine.

5. Venous Symptom Complex

The following fact is the cause of failure of the venous circulation: The ether body in the metabolic region is not sufficiently stimulated by the submerged astral body to suck the blood back again into the heart, and the etheric body cannot develop enough levity. The blue blood and also other parts of the fluid organism fall too much into *gravity*. *Blood pressure* is usually *too low*. Enlarged *varicose veins*, *hemorrhoids*, and even *leg ulcers* are formed. The ether body, not sufficiently stimulated by the astral body, becomes vegetative; indeed, it inclines toward the mineral, the stagnating blood may coagulate, and the *danger of an embolism* arises.

Here, too, as in the case of patients with disturbed circulation, all massages are carried out *carefully*, entirely *without swing*, only gradually enhancing the intensity. One begins again with the back, emphasizing the lower region, loosening and warming the whole hip region. Then only the thigh with treatment of the fascia lata and the region of the trochanter and later the calf (if at all) is added with soft suction grips.

Meanwhile the leg may be etherically enlivened through intensive but not streaming arm massages (pentagram relation). In this case we recommend bringing down upon the back the lemniscatic conclusion of the streams from both arms. Deep, soft *abdominal massages* are important in the treatment of venous disturbances. They have to be introduced early with thoroughly carried out *abdominal upstrokes*. The emphasis of all grips that have the *sartorius* as leading muscle acts in the same sucking sense, especially in its upper part. It is even possible to influence beneficially the healing and the pains of an ulcus cruris (lower leg ulcer) through improvement of the blood supply with soft sucking grips on the calf above the ulcer, and in addition, through light, circular loosening of the usually tense region around the ulcer quite gently with the flat fingertips.

It goes without saying that this treatment was preceded by the treatment of the diverting paths, thigh, hip, and abdomen.

Finally, it must be emphasized that in all venous disturbances liver rubbing is indispensable, since the liver as a large organ collects the venous blood of the entire abdominal space and leads it on to the heart. The addition of a few kidney rubbings may be helpful because in all venous congestions the so called 'kidney radiation' is too weak. The kidney, as already described, has the task of radiating the astral body into the whole region of metabolism and there to stimulate the ether body. One might also think of *heart rubbing* because it has to receive all the venous blood. Whether heart and kidney are to be included in the treatment is to be decided by the physician.

6. Sleep Disturbances

Sleep disturbances are basically rhythm disturbances of the character of respiration. Ordinary breathing is a light binding and loosening of the astral body from the physical-etheric bodies. Waking and sleeping are a longer breath. The astral body withdraws from the nerve-sense system and in the morning again dives down into it. The longest breath is dying and being born again, when a total loosening and new connection occurs.

In the *breathing process*, in its finest ramifications, are hidden the *healing forces of man*. It permits the embodiment of soul and spirit in an earthly body and holds it in the middle between too firm and too loose a tie to the physical- earthly, health being the result of this balance.

Sleep was considered holy, as a healer of the troubles of the day. In sleep the breaking down processes which are the basis of waking consciousness are equalized. It cures the sick nerve system.

The longest breath, dying and rebirth, is a grace of God like the breath, for this long breath of destiny heals the errors of one life through the balancing deeds of the next life.

The breath movement of the astral body can best be represented through a lemniscate as already described at the beginning of this book.

If upper and lower functions are balanced, sleep, too, will be healthy. One sees at once that there are two constitutional possibilities for sleeplessness.

If the nerve-sense processes predominate, the astral body being active in breaking down during waking consciousness, if acids and salts are not properly secreted (uric acid especially), then the upper astral body remains stuck in the nerve-sense system and, in order to be released, it first must dive down into the ether body where it receives the impulse for loosening.

These over-excited, over-wakeful patients must, by means of very rhythmical and warm upper arm and back massage, be brought to an improvement of the upbuilding processes of the lower man. Besides this, lower back and hip region, legs and abdomen must also be treated in order to loosen and warm the lower man in such a way that the breath may dive down deeper, thus receiving the impulse for loosening. It becomes clear that there is no one-sided treatment of the upper or lower man.

If, on the other hand, there is an inclination in the astral body and ego not to have enough interest in the incarnating dipping down, then the astral body, pictorially speaking, gets caught in the cosmos. There are human beings who do *not sleep* because they *are never properly awake*, they usually show signs of *lability*, anemic debility and similar conditions. In such cases one begins at once with stronger treatments of calf and foot, then the whole back is treated intensively downward in order to permeate the body gradually and increasingly with more consciousness.

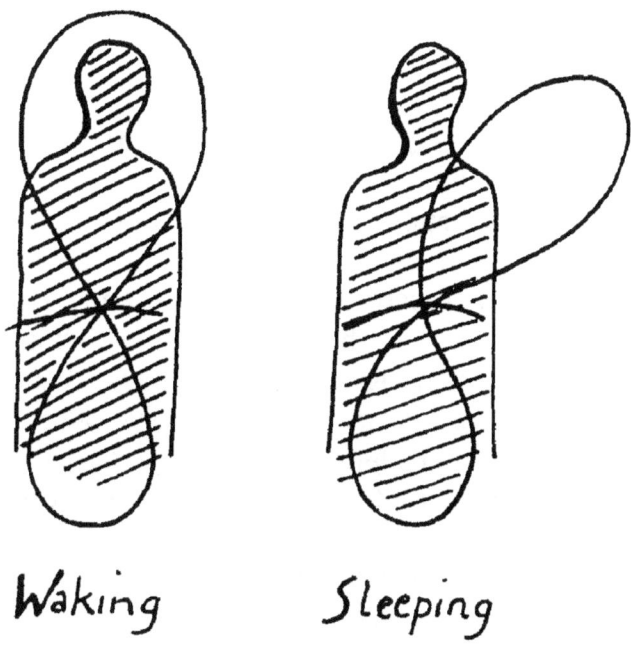

Waking   Sleeping

These are the two polar sleep hindrances. Since breathing and the rhythmical human being in general follow all soul stirrings of man, there are many psychic causes for sleeplessness. Since in most cases they are depressive soul contents, the treatment comes close to that of asthma. It will be necessary to treat the upper abdomen, lower back, and hips in order to pull down deeper the arrested breath. *Down strokes on the solar plexus*, carried out very gently, are especially effective.

In such cases it is not the task of the masseur to carry out psychotherapy. The correct attitude is silence during the massage. What has to be said can be done before or afterward. Rudolf Steiner once stated that the sensations of sympathy and readiness to help, indeed, love itself, have to be transformed into *careful technique*. The patient then feels himself secure and understood, even much better than if he is bothered with unnecessary and unsolicited counsel. The normal and humanly warm relationship between patient and masseur can be greatly improved through such an attitude.

7. Headaches of Various Origins

The head organization ought mainly to contain sense-nerve activity, some rhythmical, but very little metabolic activity. In migraine we have a flooding of the head region with metabolic life activity, an encroaching of the lower organization on the upper one. The life body with its activities is getting blocked in the head region and draws in too deeply the astral body and the ego organization. The congestion produces painful, mostly spastic processes in the head circulation.

We have found in our practice that treatment of many cases of obstinate headaches of the most varied origin with *diverting massages* has surprisingly quick results.

The two great *outstream regions* are, on the one hand, the stream from the front of the head over the crown of the head backward and down into the back. (In ancient, still-clairvoyant cultures this stream was made visible in the crest of the helmet). The other stream leads from the crown of the head over the ears into the upper arms. Both streams are especially taken care of in treatment. The cause of the congestion lies today frequently in the region of the spinal column without the patient necessarily having to suffer from back pains. Naturally, there may be various causes. In any case, a proper dosage of *diverting neck massage*, is helpful with special elaboration of these two downstream regions. Simultaneously, through strong *calf kneadings* and *foot treatments* with special attention to *ankle and heel region* one must draw the higher members deeper into the metabolic limb region. Success will depend on the proper amount of treament. In most instances, short treatments in the beginning with emphasis on calf and feet have proved beneficial. This is followed by making the back permeable and only finally by treatment of neck and head. Here occasional *loosening of the entire scalp* is helpful. Special care is to be taken of the downstrokes.

The special head massages, shown initially by Dr. Wegman herself, are recommended for patients with pale complexion, dullness in the head through over-exertion and an excessive breakdown process in the nerve-sense system. At the same time patients complain of deficient excretion. After diverting neck massages, this treatment of the head is introduced. Thereby, the blood supply of the head region is improved, the fine deposits are returned into the stream and the spasms are released. Already during the treatment the patient begins to breathe more deeply. Care is taken to improve excretion through leg and abdominal treatment and possibly kidney rubbing, and the entire downstream region from head to back is treated.

If one has the impression that disturbances in the region of the spinal column prevent the downstreaming of the forces from the head, a special *lemniscatic treatment of the spinal column* is to be recommended, especially right and left of the spinal processes, providing a better blood supply in the tissues and permeating them with consciousness. All grips must be carried out without swing, very plastically, and at the same time sucking and lifting off.

8. Constipation

In *constipation*, be it spastic or atonic, we always find that the rhythmical function of man's higher members cannot unfold in the metabolic region. In spastic constipation the astral body is cramped up; in atonic constipation also the ego organization is fettered to the physical. It will always be a question of loosening the higher members to a certain degree. This needs a careful treatment of the entire region of hip and abdomen, together with massage of the lower back and legs. The abdominal massages have to be especially thorough and intensive. The frictions and vibrations serve the activation of peristalsis and must be firmly introduced. In order to stimulate and enliven, neck massages are carried out, the effect of which according to the law of polarity radiates in front downward. Special attention is to be paid to thorough treatment of the sacrum with intensive frictions in the region between the iliac crest and the lumbar spinal column and deep kneading of the gluteus muscles. The treatment of the lower back forms the conclusion in every back massage. Regular rubbings of spleen and liver belong to the treatment of constipation.

9. Rheumatic Diseases

It is not possible to describe general courses of treatment for *rheumatic diseases*. They rest upon various metabolic disturbances and require treatment in the most varied stages. The acute inflammatory stages often slowly pass over into chronic, partly chronic sub-acute, or mineralizing, stiffening, and even deforming, forms.

Inflamed joints receive, if at all, only diverting treatments, not at the place of the illness. Only after the subsidence of the irritation symptom can the affected joint be treated. The cases of *hardening* and deformation are first treated generally with *permeating rhythm*. Thereafter the affected region is specially *loosened* and, above all, treated with warming, soft sucking grips, remaining on the same spot and thereby producing a slight *hyperemia*. A lifelessly cold part, however, is again joined to the living circulation through a streaming treatment of the whole region. Since there exists a *weakness of excretion* for such break-down products as uric acid and other irritants, one may try to stimualte this excretion through alternating organ rubbings of liver and kidney. Special organ rubbings may only be carried out by a physician's prescription.

In *mobilizing stiff joints* we must not use force. This would have a retarding effect. Enlivening, warming treatments are more effective, especially the generously applied lemniscatic treatment. In this connection,the knee plays a special role. Inflammatorily swollen and painful knees can be treated like a sprain above the knee in sucking motions. Soon thereafter one will be able to lead the stream upward in circular motion through the hollow of the knee, and gradually, by light lateral kneading and lateral lemniscates, the congestion will be loosened.

Damage to the articular cartilage of the knee also is treated by lemniscatic motions. If there exists simultaneously a relaxation of the capsule and constant danger of luxation, the knee is first strengthened by careful frictions on the guidelines of the basic form.

10. Periarthritis of the Shoulder Joint

Since we have to do here with a very painful inflammation, we employ in the acute state a *diverting* treatment with deep soft grips of the calf starting from the opposite pole; i.e., the *crossed* limb. Above we begin with light, loose back massages while sitting and the warming and loosening of the root of the limb. When the pains subside, we pass over to a *diverting neck massage* and introduce a special shoulder treatment which includes the upper arm and the arm pit. Diverting grips of the calf are continued. Only gradually may we risk a total arm massage. The emphasis remains with divertion and loosening. Later on, the joint is connected with its surrounding through lemniscates in every direction.

In this treatment, which must be carefully done in order to prevent further inflammations, it is important to adapt the quality of the grip to the stage of the illness. *Exercises to obtain mobility* must not try to loosen adhesions by force. Preferable are *swinging exercises, curative eurythmy and heat treatments* such as hayflower compresses and Fango. Mobility is often improved through Rhythmical Massage alone.

Conditions are made worse by soul burdens; indeed, they may even have been the causes of the illness. Often it becomes necessary so to treat the patient that he becomes entirely permeated by rhythm in order to produce a better body-soul balance. Human beings who with grimly persistent energy must carry out what actually is beyond their strength, are inclined to such and similar diseases in which the astral body, pictorially speaking, doggedly holds fast to a particular part of the body.

11. After-treatment of Fractures

Limbs that after a prolonged fixation have lost the connection with the total organism will slowly have to be brought back again into circulation, warmth organism, and metabolism.

We begin, therefore, to vitalize the *root of the limb* at the trunk, starting from the back, slowly descending to thigh or upper arm with warming, sucking, rhythmical grips of the basic forms until it is possible gradually to massage the whole limb. In between we introduce *massages of the back* and light *exercises of motion*. Through warming and renewed blood supply the ego organization is able to enter again. Thereby the healing of Sudeck's atrophy is aided which is a trophic disturbance in the bone showing in x-ray as a faded image and equalling a structural disturbance caused by insufficient ego presence. Here, too, through observation of the pentagram stream, one can bring in forces from the crossed limb by massaging it, not diverting as for inflammations, but leading in, that is to say, gentle streaming toward the heart. In order to *reintegrate the limb* the *lemniscatic connection* of trunk with limb and of the individual parts among themselves is of special importance and effectiveness.

The diverting treatment of *luxations and contusions* is a specially rewarding field of Rhythmical Massages. For better and faster absorption of effusions of blood it is possible to begin directly after the accident with sucking, absorbing grips above the effusion, leading the streams to the trunk. If this is repeated daily with the limb in elevated position, much pain can be avoided and bring about an astonishingly quick restoration of mobility. This is particularly the case if in the beginning compresses with pure essence of Arnica (Wala or Weleda) are added to the treatment, to be diluted more and more later on.

12. Neuritis

In the acute state of the peripheral inflammation of the nerves any general massage is contra-indicated.

The law of polarity of the upper and lower astral body joined with the law of the pentagram for the etheric body permits in this method a pain-alleviating intervention through a strongly sucking, not streaming, but localised *diverting treatment of the crossed limb*. Sciatica in the right leg, for instance, is treated in the left arm. In most cases both arms are treated, in the above case the right arm very superficially, the left arm emphatically from the upper arm downwards.

In progressive improvement of sciatica the further treatments are carried on, not in a streaming but in a gently sucking quality of grip, from inside outward. *No effleurage*. After the first purely diverting treatment there follows slowly the back treatment, very carefully downward, and soft *abdominal massages* with *upstrokes* and *liver rubbing*. Later on, the hip region is partially and gradually completely treated, and finally the sick limb. The latter, through pain and care, has more or less fallen away from the general life connection and must gradually be reunited with it. The reuniting consists in the final joining of the various parts through the lemniscate: back and hip, hip and thigh, thigh and calf.

The pauses between treatments which at first may be very short will be determined by observation of the effects. Neuritis in other parts of the body is to be treated accordingly.

13. Poliomyelitis and Paralysis of Other Causes

Poliomyelitis is a virus infection and leaves behind a peripheral, *flaccid paralysis*.

Since in the acute state it requires absolute rest, only the remaining phenomena can be treated. What we have to deal with in flaccid paralysis has been explicitly described in the chapter on the muscle system. We have to endeavour again to bring to activity the higher members of man's being fettered to the physical.

Dr. zur Linden, who is to be considered a specialist in the treatment of poliomyelitis, having developed a successful new treatment, recommends Rhythmical Massage after the subsiding of the acute phenomena, two to three times a week in connection with exercises in active motion. The latter, according to our experiences, are effective even if at first they can only be intensively visualized. Special attention has to be paid to the *keeping warm* of the paralyzed limbs. The massage itself employs thoroughly plastic grips and strives for good local blood supply. "Any rough treatment is strictly forbidden" (Dr. zur Linden). The massage is applied to the paralyzed limb and all parts that join it to the trunk. The back as central region is included in all treatments right from the beginning and later on repeatedly. In such cases it is also possible to try to supply forces to the sick region through a streaming treatment of the crossed limbs in the sense of the pentagram.

Paralysis through *apoplexy* which is caused by illness of the vascular system and appears secondarily, must be viewed differently. Poliomyelitis usually strikes young people whereas apoplexy is an illness of old age. One has to do here with a brittle, fragile, vascular system. Therefore, all massage treatments are to be carried out gently and not streaming, but carefully locally warming and stimulating. One starts from the back by vitalizing the root of the sick limb, descending over upper arm, lower arm to the hand or over the leg to the foot. The relaxed and slightly bent position, the fingers stretched out or the sole of the foot supported, is most important. Abundant rest is necessary after each treatment. Here, too, the visualized movement of the exercises is especially effective.

If the patient at the same time suffers from constipation, a light abdominal massage with liver rubbing is indicated.

14. Degenerative Illnesses of the Nervous System

In *degenerative illnesses of the nervous system*, whether they are primary or a secondary final state after inflammatory episodes, we have always to do with a *dying off process of the nerve cells*, a shrinking process with *sclerosis*. The building up processes of the nervous system, weak as they are, succumb completely. Parts of the nervous system become too dense, as it were, too physical, they pose hindrances to the higher members of man's being, causing them to lose control of the organism. In detail the processes are, naturally, complicated and differ greatly in the various forms of illness. But they are mostly treated because disturbances of motion are prevalent, beginning with the trembling of the limbs, followed by spastic-ataxic forms of movement, leading to paralysis.

In *Parkinson's disease*, for instance, one can through special rhythmical and loosening treatment of the extremities alternating with back and abdominal treatment, increase the general vitality and thereby calm the limbs. One does not use firm kneading grips but gentle uplifting kneading. The ego organization can, as far as still possible, be drawn in again through a lemniscatic back treatment.

In *multiple sclerosis* with its many changing disturbances of motion such as inhibitions, spasms, and other painful sensations at the most varied places, one will attempt to permeate the whole body with rhythm, paying special attention to the *warmth organism*. The ill person has often little understanding for the latter and can tolerate cold and draft without noticing it; indeed, in some cases even loving it. Also here one has to attempt to draw in the ego organization which needs the basis of warmth through special consideration of the lemniscatic back treatment. On the other hand, soft, deep abdominal massages as well as liver and spleen rubbings are helpful in stimulating warmth production and loosening the manifold spasms. The patients almost always suffer from chronic constipation as do all spastics.

15. Treatment of Cancer Patients

The development of cancer is a process often lasting for many years before a tumour manifests. It cannot be the task of this book to describe the physiological-anatomical drama of tumour formation with its psychic pre-stages. We can only consider the main features that give cause to a treatment with Rhythmical Massage.

Rudolf Steiner called cancer the *formation of a sense organ at the wrong place.* The genuine sense organs are formations belonging to the nerve sense system, partly pushed forward toward the periphery in order to open themselves to the influences of the outer world, and partly perceiving as hidden senses the inner states of one's own body.

All four members of man's being participate in the building up of a sense organ; then, however, the higher members, ego, astral body, and partially even the ether body, withdraw from the formation so that under certain circumstances the organ resembles a merely physical structure. That is the reason one can for instance compare the eye to a camera obscura, the ear to a musical instrument. In the nerve sense system the ether or life body, being the bearer of the growth processes, has been weakened through the ego organization to such a degree that no growth takes place, but the ether body can freely serve the process of perception. If, however, in the metabolic region islands arise from which the higher members have withdrawn, as is the case in the sense organs, and the rest of the ether body is lacking the formative power of the ego organization and the permeating breath through the astral body, then a wild growth can arise. It goes without saying that in the individual case the process is very complicated, but the processes described above explain sufficiently that the new formation cannot be that of a proper organ since it presents suffocated tissue, a kind of island of cold, having fallen away from the warmth organism; that is to say, from the control of the ego. The entire *process* is one of *involution*, frequently accompanied by *depressions* causing the patient inwardly to withdraw from the world, in the feeling of being unable to cope with life. Often one can observe an *increasing anxiety, lack of movement*, and a kind of *aphonia* which shows that the spirit-soul element no longer fully permeates the bodily senses and what goes beyond them. Certainly, according to the temperament the whole process may be overlaid and hidden. Nevertheless, it takes place in the depths. The treatment, also medication, aims to loosen the congestion and return the isolated region into the healthy life connection. One tries to attain this by leading the higher members of man into the organism via *warmth formation* and by *permeating the tissues with breath* through *mistletoe* as remedy. This expresses very roughly what is a very complicated process in the individual case.

Rhythmical Massage is, already in the psychic pre-stage, a great help. But also later on, when a manifest tumour is already present, it can be used in order to permeate the whole physical body with warmth and breath, for it relives essentially the fluid interplay of the members of man's being. Its significance becomes especially manifest when after operations and radiation treatments the affected region is to be returned again into the general life organism. Also the ill-famed *lymphatic congestions* after breast operations can be beneficially influenced through treatments leading off into the back. Here the quality of the grip that is to stimulate the plastic forces of the etheric body is of decisive importance. Since, for instance, the clearing out of the axilla (armpit) totally disturbs the lymphatic stream, we must enliven the periphery through strongly sucking grips from the root of the limb and try to lead the lymphatic streams over into the trunk along the edges of the muscles and the front and back of the armpit. Besides the enlivening work with the tips of the fingers the lemniscatic connection of arm and trunk play an important role.

Thus in the treatment of cancer, according to its stage, Rhythmical Massage may be carried out from time to time. All treaments must be careful and, above all, not streaming but locally sucking, permeating the bodily region to be massaged with consciousness. Then one can be sure that no tumour growth is stimulated and the equilibrium of the usually labile circulation is not disturbed.

In the textbooks *tumors* are described as a *contra- indication*. This is certainly justified, for the region of the tumour itself, be it benign or malignant, must under no circumstances be treated. Especially if the tumor is in a state of decomposition any massage is contra-indicated. Pre-stages and beginning tumors and post-operative cases may be treated.

16. Rhythmical Massage in Curative Education

Experience has shown that in curative education, which deals with the pliable organism of children so capable of reaction, Rhythmical Massage is an essential curative factor.

The expression *'in need of soul care,'* which Rudolf Steiner has coined for these children, can show us the way. The soul body, out of which the conscious soul part lifts itself, ensouls also the body and controls with the ego organization the bodily functions.

In curative education we have to do with children whose incarnation process was disturbed. This can take on the most individual forms and degrees, from slight soul-inhibitions to the most serious physical deformities.

Here the magic word would be *'to bring about breathing.'* For we incarnate ourselves via the breathing process right into its finest ramifications. The work of human development is carried out by the higher members of man's being themselves, one must only smooth the paths for the child by which the activity of astral body and ego unfolds in two directions, in consciousness and in movement. If one locally attracts the higher members through gently making conscious the not properly ensouled and shaped limbs or bodily parts, many a deformation can still be brought near to normal. The individuality entering the child's body has during the first seven years to *come to terms with the inherited body*.

The inherited body may be partially too dense; it must be loosened to make it possible for the soul body to dive down, immerse itself completely. It may be that the higher members have no inclination to dive down. Then, through producing a stronger consciousness especially in the back and in the legs and feet, we must bring about a stimulus for incarnation. An incarnation treatment begins in the back with a strong downward tendency, emphasizing the lower back, and continuing the downward movement to the calves of the leg and the feet. In between this the thigh and abdomen are treated. The basic form 'leg from behind' may be repeatedly used later on. The grips are soft, deep, and sucking. The lower man is above all to be permeated with breathing consciousness.

For better permeation with breath and warmth, massage treatment of all *rachitic deformities* has been successful, also the treatment of other *curvatures* and *obstructions of growth* in the limbs which often have an intrauterine origin through circulatory disturbances or strangulation.

Furthermore, *constipation in infants* is a rewarding field of treatment, likewise the dehydrating nutritional disturbances, the failure to thrive, where the gentle vitalizing of the periphery is carried out with milk rather than oil in order simultaneously to improve nutrition. The incarnation treatment has proved especially successful with children suffering from enuresis. They do not completely possess control over the lower man. Here massage of the abdomen is to be followed by a few quiet abdominal upstrokes. Also the restless children, the *'jumping jacks,'* do not dip down with their spirit and soul into the organism, in order to calm down. They have, therefore, difficulties in going to sleep. If we draw them in more deeply, they become calmer and are by themselves able also to sleep in the evening.

With older children the treatment of posture damages is to be added and in children of school age that of the various headaches. We cannot set up a scheme. The treatment of little children demands a real understanding of the stages of man's development and of the possibility of smoothing the paths for the higher members through warm, breathing and plastic grips, for the possibility of permeating it vitally, ensouling it with breathing, shaping it spiritually, and, finally, harmonizing the whole.

17. Rhythmical Massage in Psychiatry

Even in curative education there are border cases that must be called psychiatric. In psychiatry, therefore, Rhythmical Massage plays a quite similar role since the age of the patient plays a role not so much for indication but for the kind of treatment, for the quality of the grip, and so forth.

Considerations concerning human soul life, both healthy and ill, are put upon a new basis through Spiritual Science. The soul faculties of thinking, feeling, and willing rest upon the three great functional domains of the bodily processes. They unfold in close connection with processes of the body while the individual is young. Just as a blossom develops out of the purely vegetative processes of a plant whose growth metamorphoses itself into the blossom process, so soul life awakens through various stages of consciousness to an ever wider scope and deeper possibilities, borne by forces of the ether body, that free themselves by stages of the organic processes and serve the life of the spirit.

In the pamphlet *The Education of the Child in the Light of Anthroposophy* Rudolf Steiner describes this development and the magic words for education in the first three seven-year periods. They are for the first seven years: *Imitation* and *example* (proper growth of the organs), for the second seven years: *authority based on eagerness to follow* for the development of conscience, the lasting habits and inclinations that are anchored in the ether body. Here the life of feeling and sensation must be developed through awakening of the sense for beauty. Only after puberty in the third seven-year period may the child's *own judgment* be demanded and an abstract world of thought be fostered. The body, however, in its functional threefoldness is the basis of healthy soul life. The body is the mirror of soul and spirit. In the case of the so-called mentally ill, it is not the spirit that is ill, but the mirror is distorted.

We live in an age in which the breaking down nerve-sense processes dominate from the very beginning through the intellectualization of ever earlier stages of life, through the predominant interest in mechanics and the lacking education of feeling and will.

This brings about the most varied congestions of soul life in all three systems. The impressions cannot be transformed into an adequate expression acquired through the working of the ego. For *impression* and *expression* relate in the life of soul like *inhalation* and *exhalation* in the rhythmical man. Today, these two soul faculties are often not at all in balance. The impressions produce a kind of soul asthma with the danger of soul suffocation; on the other hand, unrestrained pursuit of pleasure.

Also here Rhythmical Massage can be very helpful in the many evolutionary disturbances of the soul. In all disturbances we are almost always confronted by the *lacking of a center* which cannot keep the balance between the forces of sympathy and antipathy, between surrendering to the world in bliss or confronting its loneliness and pain.

Often we have to deal with the consequences of incarnation disorders and the resulting partial excarnation processes. From all that has been presented here it might become clear that we have in Rhythmical Massage an effective method of treatment by which the binding and loosening of man's higher members may to a certain degree be furthered and harmonized if its possibilites are really employed by a knowing hand.

24.

THERAPEUTIC TECHNIQUE

In recapitulation let us once more realize that massage is an individual curative treatment which needs the complete dedication of the masseur's personality, as is the case in all curative professions. Self-discipline plays a great role. I do not intend to speak here of 'professional ethics' in the ordinary sense but of the careful techniques into which, as I have described, the feeling values have to be transformed. Naturally, the feeling values as such remain in existence, but they do not manifest in the foreground, outwardly.

The first rule is the *care of the living instrument, the hand*. Its surface should be without wound or roughness (after washing dry thoroughly), and the nails must not project beyond the finger tips. Besides the wedding ring no jewelry should be worn.

A special chapter will be devoted to the significance of the hand.

In the masseur's clothing it is important that the smock is fully closed in front and the sleeves are half or at best three-quarter length.

The masseur himself should have a good outer attitude, quiet, considerate, and determined. He needs a certain maturity in order to be able to cope with all kinds of incidents. At the outset it is good if he forms for himself a *quiet judgment about the general disposition of the patient*, regards him as a totality and only then considers the special needs. The physician's prescription does not free him of the duty of arriving himself at a clear picture of the situation, for very often he must, within the scope of the medical prescription, make independent decisions. During treatment he will always keep at a certain distance from the patient; the movements *flow out of the upper arm* which is, as in eurythmy, lifted out of gravity. In spite of this, very forceful grips may be carried out, but his own body weight must never participate.

During treatment attention has to be paid to a secure and comfortable position of the patient. Until massage begins the patient remains completely covered, and also later on, because of the importance of the warmth organism, only the region that is being treated is uncovered, but this region must not be too small. After the treatment the patient is again covered up at once. Under no circumstances may there be an open window or even a draught in the room.

Furthermore, care has to be taken that the patient does not have to look into the light, for any dazzling prevents complete relaxation.

The individual treatment must have a *structure* that has been *thought through*, possibly without repeated changes in position, so that a certain calm holds sway over the whole. After every treatment the patient has to *rest*, well covered up, at least *for 20 minutes*. Women are not treated during the period of menstruation. The duration of a treatment cannot be fixed schematically. On the average it will last for twenty to thirty minutes; in general we can say that a massage should be rather too short than too long.

The most important thing is the care and quality of the grips. Since movements relate to the fluid man, in which the life body governs the processes, also the grips ought to transform themselves into each other in a fluid continuity, and the treatment form an organic whole. Through rhythm and the gentle changes in tempo the whole assumes a musical quality. If one intends to create warmth one will, quite naturally, accelerate the successive grips but never hasten; and this acceleration will later on consciously lead back to rest.

If the full attention of the masseur is directed to his activity, a certain concentrated atmosphere spreads out as if of itself, and a diverting conversation during massage is prohibited by the very nature of the matter. If, however, the patient speaks out of inner necessity, one must not excite him through constant silence. Here the tact of the heart must find the right measure. All indications in this chapter are not dogmatic prescriptions but are meant to call into consciousness questions of which one is not always aware.

25.

THE HAND

C.G. Carus in his book *Symbolik der menschlichen Gestalt (Symbolism of the Human Figure)* begins the chapter about the hand as follows:

"With this word (the hand) we open one of the most extraordinary chapters of the entire symbolism of the human figure, for in this wondrous member there rests such an architectural profundity, its evolution shows such a strange history, its influence upon the elevation of the human soul to spirit perfection is so tremendous, that it not only gave to the researcher at all times abundant food for thought, but that apart from its special significance for the uniqueness of the person, it has long ago become a special symbol for religious and public life of peoples . . .

"We beg, command, threaten, and take an oath with the hand, a handshake obliges (binds ego to ego). We ask for the hand of a maiden. In Buddhist temples we find about a hundred different positions of hands and fingers, each of which coresponds to a definite form of prayer. We bless with the hand, we put our hand on our heart in asseveration, we raise it to heaven in solemn promise."

All these are expression that have to do with our innermost personality, with our individuality. Herder, the contemporary of Carus, also speaks significantly on the hand, stating that it is a formation full of delicate feelings and of thousandfold organic exercise. This last remark especially points to the fact that with the hand man's spirit performs acts on the physical plane, in the realm of matter, which transform the world. Just as the human spirit without matter in spiritual exercise, that is to say, in concentration and meditation, acquires new faculties, so the hand with the same perseverance practises until it has learned a new faculty, a new art.

If we say (in German) that something has 'hand and foot' we mean thereby to state that before the thinking reason, it passes as useful for the earthly plane. The hand and also the foot are on different planes a special expression of our 'humanity' distinguishing us from any animal. Even in the most highly developed ape, despite the similarity of the outer form, neither hand nor foot reach the pure relationships of measure among the parts which the human spirit imprints upon them.

In her lecture at the opening of the nurses' conference on April 30, 1970 in the Ita Wegman Clinic at Arlesheim, Switzerland, Dr. MP. van Deventer described the nature of the hands against the background of mankind's evolution as established by Rudolf Steiner in his book, *An Outline of Occult Science,** and in other publications of his.

"Hands and arms belong to the limb system of man but they play a special role in it. In the primeval past of mankind's evolution they were used as limbs like the legs for a swimming-hovering locomotion. At that time the human body was formed of finer substance, it was a kind of "fire-cloud," but inwardly alive and organized, already bearing a human shape.

When the moon left the earth and mineral substance was deposited into the human body, the gradual process of gaining an upright position began and the hands were freed from the physical earth. They became tools for the spiritual man and entered the service of the gradually developing thinking. Everything that appeared in the course of time as human culture was created by the hands. Much later the time arrived when hands and arms were adjusted to the rhythmical system. They became expression of the life of feeling in their gestures and accompany speech with expressive movements. This transition is seen most clearly in the fourth post-Atlantean cultural epoch, in Greek art where the sculptures are formed out of the individual soul and the stereotype positions of the limbs no longer predominate as was the custom in ancient cultures and traditions. In Rome we see this transition in the gesture of judgment when the Caesar pardons or condemns the conquered gladiator and expresses this with his thumb. Judging is the innermost activity of the human soul. The way this third stage of the function of arm and hand comes to expression is characteristic for the difference between Greeks and Romans. The hands will have arrived at their true task only if they, out of the rhythmical nature of man, will be streamed through by the Christ Principle, and thus will transform outer life and the world.

We see in the development of the hands a continuous process of liberation and can feel why Rudolf Steiner called them 'the most beautiful symbol of freedom'."

Thereby the hand is characterized as the most human organ, for physiologically it permits us to recognize through it much of the innermost being of man. It is especially the gestures, the way we shake hands, and many other involuntary movements that disclose much of our character, often more than we like. The individuality shapes and suffers destiny and so the traits from our past imprint themselves in the lines of our left hand, whereas those of our right hand point to the future.

---

*   Rudolf Steiner Press, London, 1979.

If we observe the whole threefold arm, we become aware of the fact that its parts carry the character of the higher members of man's being. The formation of the upper arm shows the unifying force of the ego. Only in the human being the upper arm is released from the trunk (see drawing on following page) and is movable in every direction. The ape is a degenerated counter-evolution of the human shape (See Dr. H. Poppelbaum, *Man and Animal*.) Therefore the apes always fall back on their 'hands.'

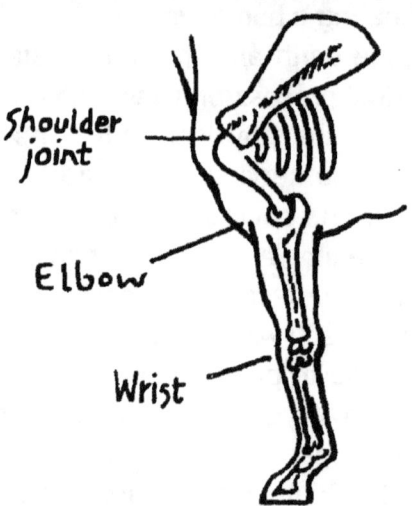

The lower arm with its two bones and the possibility of pronation and supination bears the stamp of the polarity of the astral. It is also the arm that can strike. It mirrors, right into the physical form, the possibility in the soul to turn outward or inward in the minor or major mood, to open itself and to close itself in; in short, to live in polar impulses. In man the lower arm should always be somewhat shorter than the upper arm, because this fact can prove the primacy of the spirit. If the lower arm is longer, the formation approaches the animal. In such a case one uses the expression 'monkey-arms.'

Finally, the hand, this plastic, delicately membered formation with its unheard-of possibilities of motion, shows what kind of instrument the human spirit has created for himself in order, in the realm of formative forces as used by the ether body, to be able to imitate every shape, indeed, surpassing nature to build a new world out of earthly material, the world of the arts. As we have seen, the ego imprints upon the ether body the pentagram stream. Therefore we find the pentagram also in the hand. We have pointed to this fact in the chapter, 'The Lemniscate and the Pentagram.'

A pentagram can be inscribed in the palm of the hand. We can find it as a larger or smaller one in the open hand. Its center is a special ego point; in the highest sense it is the place of stigmatization where the blood appears under the impulse of the ego.

In another way the whole human being in his functional threefoldness is depicted in the hand. The finger rays with the sensitive ends are the part in which the soul-astral element expresses itself. The point-like action belongs to the astral body and produces consciousness. The nerve-sense pole is reflected in it.

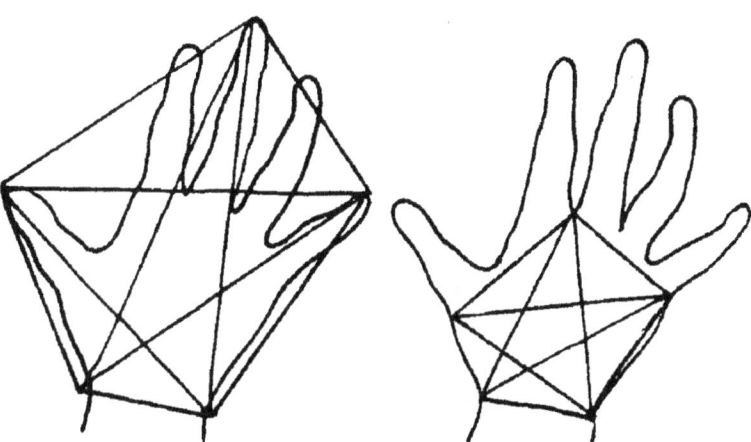

The great and small Pentagram

The palm which we can open and close, which permits us to produce systole and diastole, is related to the rhythmical system. Massage movements with the palm permit a special breathing effect. With the thumb we enter the field of the will, through the confrontation the hand becomes space. Thumb gestures are will gestures, they may have a rough, indeed, almost brutal effect. In his book *Die Hände offenbaren den Menschen (The Hands Reveal the Human Being)*, Norbert Glas, M.D. gives many examples for the differences in the nature of every single finger. From his presentations we may learn to recognize to what high degree the hands are truly 'all endowed.'

The scientist of the spirit, however, is able to reveal still more important aspects of the hand. Here again let Dr. Van Deventer speak:

"In the sixth lecture in *Excursus on the Gospel of St. Mark* Rudolf Steiner describes how the hands appear to the clairvoyant. 'Out of the fingers there come forth and radiate far into the surrounding space gleaming formations of the ether body that spread into space, now glimmering, weak, now stinging. If man is happy or sad, his fingers radiate accordingly; different are the rays of the back of the hand from those of the palm. For the observer of the spiritual the hand in its etheric and astral part is a glorious organ.'

Now, if the hand comes into touch with the surroundings, it enters - since matter in reality is condensed spirit - into relationship with the spirit of the surrounding world, for instance, with the element water. When the human beings wash their hands frequently, they become more sensitive for the environment; they are able, for instance 'to observe more intimately if a man with a brutal mind or a warm heart stands near him, whereas human beings who permit their hands to be dirty are actually also in life more coarse natures who erect walls between themselves and the more intimate relationships in their surroundings.' This becoming more sensitive in the good sense holds good only for the hands. Spirit and soul are in a very different relationship to the various parts of man's being. If, for instance, excessive cold water cures are taken, especially for children, an unhealthy oversensitiveness results.

Thus we have become acquainted with a capacity of perception for the moral qualities in our surroundings – enhanced through washing of the hands – a quality that appears as though instinctively."

There are statements of Rudolf Steiner that show that we possess also in arms and legs subconscious organs of perception for cosmic forces. In times gone by man still had a distinct feeling for the fact that the legs have a relationship to the forces of the earth, to the forces of gravity, and that the arms strive upward to the forces of the stellar universe and its harmonies. The Greek sculpture 'The Praying Youth' is an illustration of this fact. It shows the turning of the hands, following the soul, to the realms of the Gods, to the world of the stars, which the Greeks felt to be their home. This was the gesture of praying in almost all the cultures prior to the Mystery of Golgotha. Since the Mystery of Golgotha we no longer raise our hands in prayer to the Divine, but we fold the hands or put them side by side in order to find in ourselves the Divine, 'the I,' whose bringer was the Christ. We have a consciousness of self that can receive into itself the Christ force in order to let this divine force of love flow into our hands so that we may transform the earth, that we may heal and bless. – The hand, transforming the earth through our work, the healing hand, the blessing hand, are the result of the mood of prayer already practised in youth. The hands are the most formative, the most permeable of our organic limbs. They can change very much in the course of life. Soul and spirit that permeate them in training them, do not only form them but flow beyond them into the world as objective power of love, as blessing, as healing forces. After death the limbs, that is to say, the spirit that has flowed through them during life, become the physiognomy for our earthly deeds. They reveal the true quality of our earthly deeds. The hands, however, are also the creator of our future. Free deeds of love must transform the earth and man. In order to devote itself to this goal, the hand, radiating love, has been released from all ancient ties to become the symbol of freedom.